Stay Young, Start Now

❧ ❧ ❧

Praise for Stay Young, Start Now

Stay Young, Start Now reflects a family physician's deep sensitivity not only to the patients in his waiting room but also to medicine's social and historical context. Full of sensible advice, this book deserves a wide audience.
—Charles S. Bryan, M.D.
Chair, Department of Medicine, University of South Carolina
Author, *Osler: Inspirations from a Great Physician*

Stay Young, Start Now contains an enormous amount of data for the general public that is on the cutting edge of our knowledge of sexual function. In particular, I know of no other book for the general public that explores our new knowledge of how optimal female sexual function is dependent on the proper functioning of the cardiovascular system. I recommend it to any couple interested in lifetime sexual fulfillment.
—Irwin Goldstein, M.D.
Professor of Urology, Boston University School of Medicine

With all that we now know about human sexuality, the days when sexual function was expected to decline sharply or stop altogether with the passing years are gone forever. *Stay Young, Start Now: A Family Doctor's Guide to More Energy, Less Stress, and Better Sex* makes clear how a comprehensive program of health maintenance, along with an understanding of the body's natural changes as the years pass, can allow us fulfilling sexual relationships all the days of our lives.
—Saul H. Rosenthal, M.D.
Author, *Sex Over 40*

Stay Young, Start Now is recommended reading for those who really want to improve the quality of their life and fully enjoy the years ahead.
—Charles & Caroline Muir
Authors, *Tantra: The Art of Conscious Loving*

Other Books by Alan Bonsteel
A Choice for Our Children: Curing the Crisis in America's Schools
(With Carlos A. Bonilla, Ph.D., M.D.)
Published by the Institute for Contemporary Studies, Oakland, 1997

Stay Young, Start Now

*A Family Doctor's Guide
to More Energy,
Less Stress, and Better Sex*

※

Alan Bonsteel, M.D.

CELESTIALARTS
Berkeley, California

Copyright © 2000 by Alan Bonsteel. All rights reserved. No part of this book may be reproduced, stored in an information retrieval system, or transmitted in any form or by any means whatsoever without the prior written permission of Celestial Arts, except for the purpose of quoting brief passages in published reviews or articles.

CELESTIALARTS
PO Box 7123
Berkeley, CA 94707

Distributed in Canada by Ten Speed Press Canada, in the United Kingdom and Europe by Airlift Books, in New Zealand by Southern Publishers Group, in Australia by Simon & Schuster Australia, in South Africa by Real Books, and in Singapore, Malaysia, Hong Kong, and Thailand by Berkeley Books.

Text and cover design by Greene Design
Cover photo courtesy of Image Bank

Library of Congress Cataloging-in-Publication Data
Bonsteel, Alan, 1951–
   Stay young, start now : a family doctor's guide to more energy, less stress, and better sex / Alan Bonsteel.
      p. cm.
      Includes index.
   ISBN 0-89087-974-5 (pbk.)
   1. Middle aged persons—Health and hygiene. 2. Aging. 3. Sex. 4. Stress management. I. Title.
   RA777.5 .B66 2000
   613'.0434—dc21
                                        00-022663

Consult your physician before following any of the advice in this book. All health programs must be individualized. The descriptions of the side effects and interactions of the drugs and health supplements in this book are not intended to be complete. All brand names and product names used in this book are trade names, service marks, trademarks, or registered trademarks of their respective owners. Neither the author nor the publisher of this book is associated with any medical or pharmaceutical product or vendor mentioned in this book.

First printing, 2000

Printed in the United States of America

1 2 3 4 5 6 7 — 04 03 02 01 00

I don't age, I youthen.

— Merlin, explaining to a young Prince Arthur
how he was moving backward in time while
the rest of the world was moving forward.

❧ ❧ ❧

Contents

Acknowledgments................................. *xi*

Introduction..................................... *xiii*

1 Reinventing Yourself............................ 1
    SIDEBAR 1.1: 101 Goals to Change Your Life.............. 6
    SIDEBAR 1.2: The Reinvented Couple................... 10

2 What Are Your Risks?........................... 15
    Vascular Disease................................. 18
    SIDEBAR 2.1: Thinning Your Blood to Avoid Heart Attacks... 20
    SIDEBAR 2.2: How Much Time Do You Have?............. 22
    SIDEBAR 2.3: New Drug to Lower Cholesterol............ 26
    Cancer.. 32

3 The Unified Field Theory of Health................ 35
    Exercise....................................... 37
    SIDEBAR 3.1: Exercise Self-Assessment.................. 40
    Diet... 44
    SIDEBAR 3.2: Getting Started........................ 48

4 The Mind/Mind Connection..................... 53
    SIDEBAR 4.1: Heart Attack Risk Self-Assessment.......... 56

5 No Man Is an Island........................... 71
    SIDEBAR 5.1: Internet Use and Depression............... 73
    SIDEBAR 5.2: Americanization Can Be Bad for Your Health.. 74
    SIDEBAR 5.3: Social Support System Self-Assessment....... 78

6	**The Healing Power of Touch** 83
7	**Sexual Fulfillment in Second Adulthood**. 89
	Men's Issues (Required Reading for Women) 92
	SIDEBAR 7.1: Health Benefits of Regular Sex 93
	SIDEBAR 7.2: Viagra for Erection Difficulties 96
	SIDEBAR 7.3: Two New Drugs for Erection Difficulties 100
	Women's Issues (Required Reading for Men) 111
	SIDEBAR 7.4: Testosterone and Female Sexual Desire 115
8	**Children in Second Adulthood** 121
	SIDEBAR 8.1: Risks of Childbearing After Thirty-Five. 126
9	**Especially for Women**. 135
	Breast Cancer. 137
	Menopause and Estrogen Replacement Therapy. 139
	SIDEBAR 9.1: Two New Drugs for Women Who Can't Take Estrogen. 140
	SIDEBAR 9.2: Evista as an Alternative to Estrogen. 143
	SIDEBAR 9.3: Advice for Women Who Decline to Take Estrogen 144
	Hysterectomy. 150
	SIDEBAR 9.4: Women and Heart Attacks 152
10	**Especially for Men** 157
	Prostate Problems 157
	SIDEBAR 10.1: Prostate Cancer Prevention 158
	Heart Attack. 161
	SIDEBAR 10.2: What Is Your Health Emotional Quotient?. . . . 162

11 A Checklist of Preventive Medicine................ 165
Blood Pressure 165
Cholesterol... 166
Colon Cancer 166
Low Thyroid... 169
Diabetes.. 169
Skin Cancer 170

12 The Evidence for Health Supplements 173
SIDEBAR 12.1: The Antioxidant Revolution 175
Aspirin... 178
SIDEBAR 12.2: Homocysteine and Heart Attacks.......... 180
Omega-3 Fatty Acids 181
Garlic.. 183
DHEA 184
Melatonin.. 186
Human Growth Hormone 187

13 The Battle of the Bulge 189
SIDEBAR 13.1: 44% of Your Calories Come from This 192
SIDEBAR 13.2: 21 Ways to Lose 21 Pounds 196
SIDEBAR 13.3: Pumping Iron for Weight Maintenance...... 200
SIDEBAR 13.4: The Worst Exercise for Losing Weight 201

14 How to Avoid Doing Yourself In **203**

    Tobacco 205

    SIDEBAR 14.1: Health Effects of Smoking (Partial List) 206

    SIDEBAR 14.2: Zyban for Smoking Cessation 209

    Alcohol 212

    SIDEBAR 14.3: Health Effects of Alcohol (Partial List) 214

    SIDEBAR 14.4: ReVia for Alcoholism 218

15 Choosing Your Health Care Provider **221**

16 If You Need Surgery **235**

    SIDEBAR 16.1: Surgery for Angina and Coronary
                          Artery Disease 236

    SIDEBAR 16.2: Surgery for Back Pain 240

17 Meditation: It's Not What You Think **243**

18 When Things Go Wrong **251**

19 Does Anyone Actually Follow This Advice? **257**

20 Follow Your Dream **263**

    Appendix 1: Summary of Recommendations 266

    Appendix 2: Recommended Reading 270

    Index 277

    About the Author 286

Acknowledgments

It would be impossible to thank everyone who has helped bring this book to the public, so the names that follow omit many important contributors.

I would first like to thank my patients, who have been not just my teachers, but also my inspiration. For those many patients I have been privileged to know, I can only thank you for allowing me to share your lives, and for the courage you have so often shown in the face of adversity.

I would like to thank the many medical personnel who have been a part of our team: the nurses, the nurses' aides, the paramedics, the physical therapists, the respiratory therapists, the lab technicians, the medical transcriptionists, the housekeeping staff, and the lady who registers the patients and assures them that the doctor will be coming soon. Our medical care system wouldn't work without you, and I know that all too often you don't get the thanks you deserve.

Special thanks to the medical reviewers and consultants: Carlos Bonilla, Ph.D., M.D.; Steve Kaplan, M.D.; Ingrid Lopes, D.O.; Charles Bryan, M.D.; Saul Rosenthal, M.D.; Dean Ornish, M.D.; Lee Lipsenthal, M.D.; Steve Guffanti, M.D.; Peter Van Houten, M.D.; and Winnifred Cutler, Ph.D. Thanks also to our text reviewers, Odette Gaulin Charbonneau, Maurice Cloud, and David Barulich.

Thank you to a rural hospital administrator who encouraged me in this project and whose vision and dedication has well served his community: Charles Guenther of Eastern Plumas District Hospital in Portola, California.

Thank you to Dr. Peter Beoris of Valley Emergency Physicians for years of patient mentoring during my maturing as an emergency physician, and for his tireless work in providing quality emergency services to California's rural hospitals.

Most of all, thanks to my wife and partner in this book, Chantal Charbonneau, to whom I can only say, *Chantal, je t'aime fort.*

—Alan Bonsteel, M.D.
San Francisco, California

Introduction

We are living in an era in which our physiological and attitudinal age is at least as important as our chronological age. For those who are willing to make a modest investment in their health and to take advantage of all that we now know about staying young, it's possible to slow down the biological clock dramatically. In a few cases, such as heart disease and osteoporosis, it's even possible to *reverse* the biological clock. This book will show you how.

Stay Young, Start Now is a book that only a family practitioner could have written. You'll rarely read about us in the newspapers—generalists seldom become famous. We do very little research. We don't run renowned medical centers such as the Mayo Clinic. We rarely become deans of medical schools.

What we do is see patients, and our patients' kids. We listen to them. We treat their migraines, their high blood pressure, their gynecological problems, and their depression. We see them not just as bodies, but as people who have a psychological and a spiritual dimension.

This book has grown out of my years of work as a family practitioner—and often, as well, an emergency physician—work that has always been rewarding and frequently even moving. My years in my clinic have left me with memories of patients whose lives have touched mine and enriched me forever. I've shared their dreams, and I've been there for the milestones in their lives. I've delivered their babies and shared that joyous moment when new life is brought into this world. I've also shared their celebration when they got married and their despair when they were divorced. I've tried to be there for them at the times when I had bad news and had to tell them that things did not look good.

In my emergency room, I've had giddy victories when the medical team triumphs and death is cheated, and the patient receives the gift of another chance at life. I've also been there for the crushing defeats when we did everything we could, and still lost, and I've held the hands of my patients as the life ebbed out of them. Every day, on the Shakespearean stage of life that is my ER, I see moving stories of courage, love, and devotion.

In *Stay Young, Start Now*, I've taken what I've learned from those many years of training and experience to offer you, in language that is accessible to nonmedical people, the knowledge you need to stay youthful, mentally sharp, and with an unshakable sense of well-being.

What this book is *not* is an encyclopedia of health. You won't find anything here about psoriasis or gout or dozens of other maladies. What I have done is to arm you with the knowledge to be in the best possible overall health—in essence, to give you a framework. If you find yourself with a particular illness, there are plenty of information sources you can turn to—and you'll want to consult your health care provider in any case.

Few of us have the time to constantly obsess about our health, but it turns out that we can dramatically decrease our risks through some simple interventions. What I've done in this book is to take a look at virtually all the key health issues that you need to address to stay young, seen from the point of view of a family practitioner—a generalist physician trained to look not only at the whole body but the whole *person*. At the same time, I've condensed this information to the point that you'll actually be able to read it.

Society today is far faster paced than it once was, and that fast pace isn't just imaginary—studies have shown that people now even *talk* about 40 percent faster than they did in the early 1950s. And yet, the speed and the constant change and innovation with which we are faced may be our salvation. It is now clear that those whose minds are constantly challenged retain their mental acuity far longer in life, and that the decline in memory and mental sharpness once thought inevitable may be largely preventable.

Not only is change a constant in our lives, but the pace of that change accelerates every year. Hardly any of us holds a job or owns a business so secure that we aren't constantly looking over our shoulder to see who has a newer technology that can overtake us. Nor is changing technology by any means the only revolution transforming us. Our family lives and the way we look at our friendships and our romances have undergone great upheavals, and continue to do so.

Now we live with a dramatically higher divorce rate, and we relocate at a far greater rate than any previous generation. The stable relationships we once took for granted are a victim of that faster pace of life, and we find that we have to work at staying in touch and at having something more than the dysfunctional family that has become so common. The effect on our health and well-being is profound; there is no question that the quality of our social support system is intimately linked to our physical and emotional health. As the poet John Donne said, "No man is an island, entire of itself."*

When we were teenagers and into our twenties, we believed we were immortal. We drove fast, we free-climbed mountains, we drank hard, and we smoked. As we grow older and wiser, however, we come to realize that we're not immortal after all. Our bodies don't keep up the way they used to, and we've lost some family and friends. And yet, out of the unsettling but unsurprising realization that we are not immortal can come, paradoxically, the ability to transform ourselves and to live fully and youthfully in the moment. We have within our grasp the ability to put our fears and phobias behind us and to enjoy life to the fullest, while benefiting from knowing how to keep our bodies fit enough to maintain the pace.

As it turns out, the illnesses that are the big killers fall into only two broad categories—vascular disease and cancer—and the principles for reducing your risk of both are very similar. It turns out as well that the same interventions for reducing your risk of these two illnesses will also dramatically reduce your risk of many *other* chronic diseases. And we now know enough about the ways we do

---

*Source notes are not given in this book for anecdotal quotations from authors or works.

Introduction

ourselves in—the various addictions that are epidemic in our society—to open the door to an addiction-free life for everyone.

This book is unique in that it integrates all the factors that are important to good health and well-being. I'll be talking about the five essentials of good health: diet, exercise, a social support system, regular meditation, and an addiction-free lifestyle. Along the way, I'll talk about many other things as well: the latest advances in drugs, the changes in your sex life that come with the passing years, even the challenges of starting a second family—or a first—beyond the age at which it was once traditional. Again and again, I'll come back to the theme of how difficult—and wrong—it is to consider one aspect of our health in isolation, without looking at the whole. The further I've gone in my career as a physician, the more amazed I have become at how interrelated it all is, and at the folly of taking one organ system in isolation and trying to treat it without reference to the rest of the body.

It is also futile, in my view, to treat just the physical body without dealing with the psychological and even the spiritual dimensions of the patient's life. If there is one thing I have learned as a physician, it is that a person's sense of meaning and purpose in life is primordial. The individual who believes, as Robert Frost expressed it, that "I have promises to keep, / And miles to go before I sleep," can carry on quite nicely with a body with a few defects here and there. However, the converse is never true. I know that the lost soul with no idea what purpose is served by existing on this planet will be plagued with every malady in the book, and will be ill served with pills and injections.

I hope that this book will revolutionize your approach to your health. And I hope that, in rediscovering the dormant you, taking care of your physical body becomes not a task but a joyful realization of a newfound purpose, a natural alignment with your vision for the rest of your life.

Good reading, and here's to the best years of your life!

CHAPTER ONE

Reinventing Yourself &

I heard the whine of the air ambulance above me and felt the thrill every rural emergency physician knows when death has once again been cheated—the relief that soon my patient would be whisked away to the safety of the intensive care unit of a large urban hospital. I glanced at Steve,[*] the heart attack victim drenched in sweat on the gurney, and then at the monitor still showing him jumping from one nerve-wracking heart rhythm to another.

As the twin-turbine-powered helicopter drew closer, I heard the familiar *whup-whup-whup* of the rotor, followed by the feathering of the engines as the pilot brought his bird onto our tiny landing pad. In the hundreds of times I have called in air ambulances to the small, isolated hospitals in which I have always worked, I have never tired of that emotional moment when help descends from

---

[*] The names of all the patients in this book have been changed. Their stories, however, are true.

the sky, and we know that, barring a last-second cardiac arrest, we have kept the patient alive on our watch.

I saw the fear in Steve's eyes as he faced the unknown of something that wasn't supposed to happen while he was still in his mid-forties: a myocardial infarction, or MI. He was surrounded by tubes and dials and electric wires, the paraphernalia of the tissue plasminogen activator (TPA) we had given him to dissolve the clot in his left anterior descending artery—the "widow maker." On the other side of the gurney, his wife and three kids anxiously clung to the railing. I wish I knew what to tell families in this setting. No one knows better than I that a heart attack can degenerate at any moment into a full cardiac arrest. Unlike on TV, in the real world most cardiac arrest victims don't survive.

"The helicopter's here," I told Steve. "The arrhythmias from your heart attack and from the TPA we gave you, seem to be quieting down, and I think you're going to be OK. You'll be at the Loma Linda Medical Center in about an hour, in their cardiac intensive care unit with some superb and very caring cardiologists."

Steve nodded. "Thanks, Doc," he said. "I appreciate everything you've done."

"Steve," I continued, "I know that having a heart attack was the last thing you wanted for this nice Labor Day weekend, but maybe there's a silver lining in this after all. Maybe this will turn out to be the wake-up call you need to make the lifestyle changes you know you *have* to make. To stay out of trouble, you're going to have to revolutionize your diet and your exercise program, and, most importantly, you're going to have to ditch those cigarettes. I hate to lecture people, but you seem like such a nice guy, and I want you to do well. You're a smart man, and you have a wonderful, supportive family. You have everything going for you."

Steve nodded mutely. The jumpsuited flight nurses arrived with their gurney, and I gave them the rundown on our patient, using the alphabet-soup jargon of the medical profession. Ten minutes later, having switched monitors, oxygen tanks, and IV lines, they were pushing Steve out the door toward the landing pad, his family trailing behind.

"Wait a minute," he shouted, just as we cleared the ER doors. "Get me a wastebasket." As a puzzled nurse brought one, he turned to me and held up a pack of Marlboros.

"Doc, you see these? Watch this!" he exclaimed, throwing them into the trash. I gave him the "high five," but inwardly I wondered if he really meant it. It was a gesture I'd seen often in similar circumstances. As a motivator, fear unfortunately goes only so far.

I watched the helicopter take off and bank toward the Los Angeles basin, the downdraft of the rotor bending back the tree branches, the smell of aviation kerosene permeating the air. The towering Sierra Nevada behind Lone Pine provided a stunning backdrop for what has to be the most spectacular setting of any hospital in the United States. I allowed myself a moment to admire the clouds swirling around the summit of Mt. Whitney, and then turned toward the waiting room to face the bread-and-butter of the emergency room doc: the earaches, skinned knees, and migraines that had piled up while we treated Steve's MI. His case had been stressful, but no more so than the many medical emergencies, car-crash victims, and gunshot wounds that are also the life of an ER physician.

Within days, Steve's case had faded from my mind and joined the ranks of the two hundred or so heart attacks I have treated in my career. When he and his wife, Louise, stopped into my ER to visit me four months later, I hardly recognized him. Not only was he not drenched in sweat, but he had dropped at least twenty pounds.

"Remember me?" he asked, pumping my hand excitedly. "Doc, I want to thank you for all you did to save my life, but most of all I want to thank you for taking the time to talk to me about turning my life around. Remember how I threw away those cigarettes? Well, I never did touch another. All I could see in my mind all the time I was in the ICU was the faces of my kids watching me there in the ER, and I knew I had to do whatever it takes to be around to see them grow up. Louise and I have given up beef and pork, and we're walking together almost every night now and square dancing on Wednesday nights. It's really put the romance back in our marriage!" Louise stood by his side, beaming as she put her arm around his neck.

I hope I do deserve some small part of the credit for his turnaround, along with his cardiologist, his family physician, and his loving family. The lion's share of the credit, though, goes to Steve himself. He transformed a setback that turns some patients into cardiac cripples into the opportunity to reinvent himself.

I wish that more people could have the opportunity to reassess who they are and who they want to be without, of course, the need for that bolt out of the blue, that illness that tells them their health can no longer be taken for granted. And more and more people do seem to realize that our health is inextricably linked to many other aspects of our lives: our family life and social support system, our love life, our spiritual life, and our work and sense of meaning and purpose. Many people today are managing to reinvent themselves in ways that would have been inconceivable to previous generations.

One of my favorite soliloquies from the works of Shakespeare is his "Ages of Man" from *As You Like It:*

All the world's a stage,
And the men and women merely players;
They have their exits and their entrances;
And one man in his time plays many parts.

The stanzas of the "Ages of Man" chronicle the stages of life from infancy to youth to adulthood and old age—stages in a lifetime that in Shakespeare's era was often brutally short. As recently as a century ago, one didn't expect to be youthful at age fifty; one expected to be dead.

Until now, the roles corresponding to life's various stages seemed preordained and inevitable. Not long ago, a patient of mine named Norma told me, "By the time she was forty-five, my mother didn't just look old, she looked old and *tired.* Now I'm

SIDEBAR 1.1

101 Goals to Change Your Life

There is no question that a true paradigm shift is more desirable than incremental change, simply because incremental changes produce incremental improvements, so the results are harder to measure, harder to appreciate, and more difficult to sustain. Not only are people more likely to stick to the twin mantras of diet and exercise if they are truly strict about eating healthful foods and breaking out a sweat every day, but also embracing the whole formula of transformed relationships, overcoming stress, and leading a purposeful and fulfilling life produces such dramatic results that it is almost impossible to turn back.

For you to resolve to do a complete makeover of your approach to your health, certainly the first hurdles are in overcoming inertia and deciding where to start. It is only human, after all, to have doubts and second thoughts about whether the "new you" is really going to emerge or whether old habits will prevail.

The way to begin is to *set clear goals for yourself.* Even if you doubt whether a particular goal can be achieved, even if you can't clearly visualize the outcome you want and imagine yourself having achieved that goal, *simply setting the goals will put the process in motion.* The act of writing down your goals will put your subconscious to work in achieving them and will allow your conscious mind to visualize the desired outcomes.

So take out a piece of paper and a pencil or pen. Write down the following goals:

1. The ideal weight you would like to see for yourself.
2. The sports you would like to be able to do without getting winded.
3. The body build you would like for yourself.
4. The cholesterol level you would like to have.
5. The blood pressure you want.
6. The health issues you would like to have resolved.

7. The addictions you would like to give up: cigarettes, alcohol, whatever.

Are you finding it easier already to visualize your goals? Great!

Now I want to ask you to take an expanded view of what your health means, including all the other aspects of your life that are intimately interrelated. On the same piece of paper, write down the following goals:

1. The relationship you would like with your spouse, including the romantic and sexual life you would like to have.
2. The relationship you want with your children.
3. The relationships you want with your friends and associates.
4. The work you want to be doing.
5. The purpose and sense of meaning you want for your life.
6. The spiritual life you want.

Keep adding to this list until you run out of ideas. You may reach 101, or even more. *Be as specific as you can.* If you want to finally get the clutter in your closet organized, write that down. If you want a golden retriever that joyously greets you when you come home, write that down.

When you are through with your list, discuss it in detail with your spouse or significant other, and discuss his or her list as well. Share with each other your thoughts on what it would take to achieve those goals, as well as your fears and hesitations. Focus first on those goals that appear on *both* lists and support each other in your goals.

When you are through with your list, *don't* put it in the back of a drawer somewhere. Put it on your bulletin board or tape it to your bathroom mirror. Be sure it is in a place where you will see it often every day.

Congratulations—you've begun your journey. This list will serve you in amazingly good stead in the years to come.

the same age, and there's a part of me that buys into that same image. But there's another part of me that still has the self-image of me waiting for my date at the junior prom. And when I'm down at the health club, I can't quite keep up with the nineteen year olds, but I certainly don't look or feel like my mother did at my age."

An ice-hockey buddy of mine, Edward, had much the same story. "When my father was forty-four, he had the attitude that there were just certain things you didn't do at that age. And I guess it's no surprise that, sitting in front of the TV all the time, he really started to put on some weight in his mid-forties. Now I'm forty-four myself, and I'm mixing it up pretty good with a lot of guys in their twenties and having the time of my life."

Nor is it just a question of more knowledge about health and better medical care. One of the biggest changes in our lifestyles has been a new openness in communication, a new willingness to tell the truth about who we are and how we feel. One of the reasons that Shakespeare's ages of man seemed preordained is that people bought into those changes and adopted those roles, subconsciously or otherwise. People now can honestly say, "I'll be damned if I'm going to sit in front of the TV with my pipe and slippers like my dad did at this age," or, "I'm not yet ready to be so weighed down with life—like my mother—that I'm willing to let go of my inner child, the joyous and sometimes silly side of me." At the same time, though, they can also say, "I don't buy into the image of the surfer or the jock as my masculine ideal," or, "I'm tired of trying to live up to the image of the superwoman who has it all. I need to set my own priorities."

We have the extraordinary privilege of remaining physically and emotionally youthful far longer than previous generations, while profiting from the experience and wisdom of the passing years. Gail Sheehy, in *New Passages,* found that by age fifty the women she studied had "opened up intellectually and flowered emotionally. Their verbal fluency was higher. They had become more spontaneous, humorous, and expressive." The psychiatrist George Vaillant found that the successful men in their fifties he had studied had developed an ability to handle life's accidents and conflicts without passivity, blaming, or bitterness. As Ralph Waldo Emerson expressed it, "People do not grow old; when they cease to grow, they become old."

There was a time when we thought of the young as youthful because they were in a state of rapid evolution and change. Now we are *all* rapidly evolving, and our chronological age is becoming less and less relevant. All around us we can see people who have transformed their lives and are scarcely the same persons they once were. Not only are we living longer, but also we have the resources to make dramatic changes in ourselves. With courses and counseling and information of all sorts readily available, we are now living in a world in which we can perhaps reshape our lives with a wisdom tempered by experience.

Ironically, the opportunity for self-transformation often comes disguised as a setback—the financial failure, the relationship gone

SIDEBAR 1.2

The Reinvented Couple

I didn't know Ted and Francine in their "before" days, but they're regular patients in my practice now, and I've had some long conversations with them about their transformation.

Not too many years ago, Ted was a typical victim of middle-age spread. He tried to watch his diet, but he had gotten out of the habit of regular exercise, and each year he'd put on a few pounds. One day he was watching college basketball on TV, and something snapped.

"I was watching a postgame interview with one of the players, when suddenly I had this eerie feeling, as though I was going back in time. The player on TV looked a lot like me, back when I played intercollegiate basketball, and he had all the enthusiasm and energy I used to have. He and his team had won their game, and they were all whooping it up and giving each other the high five. All of a sudden, I had tears in my eyes. It brought back to me all the closeness I felt with my old basketball buddies, and the good times we had together. I looked down at my spare tire and I flashed on how far downhill I had gone.

"Then they put this beer commercial on," he continued, "and I got pissed off. I got off the sofa and turned off the TV. Without even thinking about what I was doing, I put on an old pair of gym shorts that barely fit, an old white T-shirt, and my tennis shoes."

Thus improbably attired, Ted shuffled out the front door for a run around the block.

"When I saw him go out the door like that, I couldn't help laughing," Francine recounts. "I mean, I know you're not supposed to laugh at your husband, but he didn't even fit into his gym clothes anymore. I thought he'd jog once, and then head right back to the TV. But the next day he went out again, and the next, and then he was talking to me about getting serious about our diet. Pretty soon, I was signed up at the gym, and we were weighing ourselves together almost every day and watching the pounds drop off."

"I never thought I'd recapture the closeness of those old days on the basketball team," Ted says, "but I got it back, in spades. I'm playing basketball every Thursday night with a bunch of guys my own age, and it's like we've mellowed with the times and can be even closer to each other than I remember from college. We don't have anything to prove, so it's not the end of the world if we lose a game. And it's not like the testosterone is flowing after the game and we need to go out cruising for chicks, like in the old days. We're really out there for each other now."

When I ask Ted and Francine how their love life is going, they're like a couple of giggly teenagers.

"Now that we've knocked off the pounds and gotten back into exercise, we have a lot more energy," Francine says. "Our love life has really taken off."

"Yeah, we've really turned back the clock," Ted agrees. "There's nothing like dropping fifty pounds to get a couple turned on to each other again. I tell all the other couples we know, 'Kill your TV, break out a sweat, turn back the clock. You won't regret it.'"

sour, sometimes even the heart attack like Steve's that tells us things will never again be the same, for better or for worse. What allows us to transcend these setbacks is the realization that they are always there for a purpose, that one door never closes without another door opening.

What very often slows us down in moving forward is the memory of our life's tragedies, our regrets, or our longing for what might have been if things had only played out differently. Yet those experiences were sent to us to teach us what we need to learn, to forge us on life's anvil into stronger steel.

What is past is prologue, not destiny, and the experience you wanted is still within your grasp. You *can* have that loving and intimate relationship you envisioned, you *can* have the business of your own you've always dreamed of, you *can* take that trip around the world.

We have a deep need to be productive and to make a contribution throughout our lives. Once people retire and cease to feel useful, heart attack and cancer rates soar. The great educator and physician Maria Montessori, after a lifetime of fulfilling work in the service of children, at the age of eighty-two was told by some of her students that she needed to slow down. She exclaimed, "What—am I no longer of use?" and only hours later, died of a stroke. More recently, the world mourned as it heard the news of the death of Charles Schulz—at precisely the moment that his final *Peanuts* comic strip appeared in newspapers. As Sigmund Freud observed, the two essential elements of happiness are to love and to work.

All of us fear risk, yet risk is what gives life its thrill and excitement. There would, after all, be no winning if not for its friend and constant companion, losing. When one of my patients tells me of his dream of doing what he always wanted, but admits to holding back because of a steady but dull job, I ask him which of two tombstones he would prefer—the one carved with the epitaph "He made a living" or the one with the message "He was himself."

We now know that we can rediscover the wonder and laughter of our inner child and that we can find the sense of adventure and risk-taking of the adolescent who still dwells within us. We know that the limitations on what we can do with our lives are primarily those we place on ourselves. And we know that true transformation—that paradigm shift that allows us to transcend the person we once were and shoot for the moon and the stars—is achievable.

We now have within our grasp an amazing gift: the ability to reinvent ourselves.

CHAPTER TWO

What Are Your Risks? ✌

The human body and spirit are truly awe inspiring. The longer I practice medicine, the more often I'm reminded of a passage from Shakespeare's *Hamlet:*

What a piece of work is man!
How noble in reason, how infinite in faculty,
In form and moving how express and admirable,
In apprehension how like a god.

In undertaking the audacious task of talking about the myriad dimensions of health, from the sublime to the ridiculous, from the philosophical to the proctological, it's hard to know where to begin. But if the body is the temple of the soul, perhaps the place to start is with the innards of the "house" we inhabit—to begin with the plumbing.

STAY YOUNG, START NOW

Now that we're old enough to have figured out that we're probably not immortal—and the "probably" is tongue in cheek!—one of the most worthwhile exercises in taking inventory of our well-being is to give some thought to what our health risks are. Obviously, the risks vary tremendously from person to person. The sedentary, overweight person is going to have vastly different risks than the Flying Wallendas, who stay in superb physical condition while taking their chances on the high wire. Everything that follows, therefore, is aimed at the mythical person in "average" health.

I quote these statistics without any great hope that, by themselves, they will be big motivators. People are rarely moved by dire warnings of future illness or death, even if delivered by the man in the white coat with all the drama of Dickens's Ghost of Christmas Future. I've long since learned, as most physicians have, that warnings of future mortality, even if believed, are not very effective. Most patients don't change their lifestyles much as a result of such warnings unless faced with their imminent demise, which often means the heart attack that gets their attention and suddenly has them listening to their physician. Otherwise, the usual reaction is, "Well, Doc, you gotta go sometime, and I'd rather be happy now than sacrifice."

What does change people's behavior is the promise of a more fulfilling life *now*—better fitness, a greater sense of well-being, improved appearance, a better sex life. "Changes need to be made not on fear of dying but on joy of living," as Dr. Dean Ornish has said.

The usefulness of confronting our risks of dying is not so much in trying to motivate people to live longer, but to live more fulfilling lives in the here and now. The truth is that the three big killers—heart attacks, cancer, and strokes—often take their time about killing, leaving people severely impaired while they undergo lingering deaths. Nonfatal heart attacks really have a way of slowing people down, often causing *congestive heart failure,* in which the heart muscle becomes stretched and flaccid and fails to pump well enough to keep the lungs and ankles from filling with fluid. Cancer, of course, is no one's idea of a quick or easy way to go. And strokes can rob us of what we value most: our mental acuity.

The *good* news is that the Big Three are largely preventable, or at least postponable. Again, that's not true for everyone; there are always going to be people like Sergei Grinkov and Jimmy Fixx, athletes who died at an early age despite having done everything right. But for most of us, most of the time, we have far more control over our health than we give ourselves credit for. And it turns out that the interventions that will decrease the risk of the Big Three are not sacrifices at all, but lifestyle changes that will lead to a more fulfilling and happier life *right now.*

In the developed countries, these three broad diagnoses are responsible for about three-quarters of all deaths. Heart attacks will kill about 35 percent of us, cancer about 30 percent, and strokes about 10 percent. *All other causes of death put together account for only about one-quarter of all fatalities.* With the advent of antibiotics, infectious diseases such as pneumonia now rarely kill, unless the patient is already weakened by cancer or some other debilitating disease. AIDS is a very serious public health problem in the United States, but, despite the impression that television viewers may get from hospital soap operas, it is not one of the big killers for those not in a risk group. We may worry about car accidents and murders, but they represent a small percentage of fatalities in this country.

Vascular Disease

Heart attacks and strokes are really subsets of the same illness: *vascular disease* (disease of the arteries and veins), which is a "disease of modern society." As recently as a century ago, heart attacks were a trivial cause of death, and they are still a very minor cause of death in underdeveloped countries. The average life span in the United States in 1900, as a result of untreatable infectious diseases such as tuberculosis, as well as high mortality in childbirth and high infant mortality, was around forty-seven, an age at which heart attacks are not yet common. People ate low-fat, high-fiber diets, they got plenty of exercise, and cigarettes had not yet become popular. Since 99 percent of human evolution has taken place under such circumstances, mostly with even shorter average life spans, our poor coronary arteries aren't "designed" to take the punishment we now give them.

Heart attacks are caused by blockages in the three small coronary arteries that deliver blood, and therefore oxygen, to the heart itself. The heart is linked to the vascular system by the "great vessels": the superior and inferior *venae cavae* (veins) leading into it, the *pulmonary arteries and veins* linking it to the lungs, and the *aorta* leading out (see Plate 3). Despite the massive amounts of blood flowing through the heart, the heart's own oxygen supply comes not from the great vessels, but rather from the pencil-thin coronary arteries that surround the heart and then dive deep into the heart muscle. When cholesterol plaques build up on the walls of the coronary arteries, the arteries become much more susceptible to the blockages that cause heart attacks. A patient whose heart chronically doesn't receive enough blood and oxygen from compromised coronary arteries develops *angina,* a severe chest pain brought on by exercise or emotional stress.

The right side of the heart receives oxygen-depleted blood from the superior and inferior venae cavae. This blood is pumped through the lungs, where it is oxygenated, and back to the left side of the heart, which pumps it to the rest of the body via the aorta. The three coronary arteries, which originate at the base of the aorta, are the right coronary artery, the left coronary artery, and the circumflex artery. (The latter two begin as the left mainstem coronary artery and then subdivide.)

The heart's pacemaker (which originates the electrical impulse that tells it how fast to beat) is the *sinoatrial node* in the right atrium (see Plate 2). The electrical impulses from this pacemaker travel to the *atrioventricular node* and are then transmitted through the two ventricles, such that the two atria beat in tandem,

> **SIDEBAR 2.1**
>
> ## Thinning Your Blood to Avoid Heart Attacks
>
> Two new studies seem to show a decrease in the rate of heart attacks as a result of two seemingly very different interventions. In the first study, one group of patients was asked to drink five glasses of water a day, while a control group continued life as usual. It was discovered that the patients drinking five glasses of water every day had a much lower rate of heart attacks.
>
> In the second study, the rate of heart attacks in people who gave blood regularly was compared to that of a control group of people who appeared to be similar to the study group in every way—except that they never gave blood. It turned out that the blood donors had a far lower rate of heart attacks.
>
> What these two approaches have in common is that they tend to lower the *hematocrit*, which is the percentage by volume of red cells in the blood. (The other component of blood is serum, which is mostly water). In a normal, healthy person, about half of the blood is composed of red blood cells.
>
> It has long been known that a high hematocrit is associated with more blood clotting—and after all, clots in the crucial coronary arteries are the fundamental cause of heart attacks. For this reason, patients with *polycythemia vera*, a condition in which the hematocrit runs high for unknown reasons, are treated by drawing off units of blood. This works because the body replaces serum faster than it replaces blood cells, thus effectively reducing the hemat-

ocrit. (The only other disease still treated by the medieval practice of bloodletting is *hemochromatosis,* a pathological buildup of iron in the blood and tissues.)

Donating blood would also be expected to reduce the risk of heart attacks because it reduces the level of iron in the blood by a small but significant amount. High levels of iron, which is an oxidant, have been correlated with higher rates of heart attacks (as well as cancer).

An obvious criticism of the blood-donation study is that people who donate blood tend to be more health-conscious than those who don't, so it is difficult to match them accurately against a control group. And part of the reason for the lower rates of heart attacks in blood donors may be the "helper's high" that results in better health—a very real, but less "scientific," explanation for the outcome.

Both of these studies were small and must still be considered preliminary. However, there are logical reasons why these two activities may help—and both are desirable in their own right. Drinking copious amounts of water has been known for at least a century to reduce the incidence of kidney stones, one of the most painful conditions known to medicine. And, as a veteran emergency physician, I have had trauma cases in which the floor of my ER ran red with blood, yet the patients lived to see the light of another day—because of the generosity of people like yourself who made the effort to donate blood.

> **SIDEBAR 2.2**
>
> ## How Much Time Do You Have?
>
> The average American can currently expect to live to age 77. To find out *your* anticipated life span, answer the following questions, and add or subtract the number of years in each item from age 77.
>
> This questionnaire is aimed at readers no older than 55. Those who have already exceeded that age can anticipate an even longer life span.
>
> 1. ***Sex:*** Female—add 2 years to 77. Male—no change.
> 2. ***Genes:*** Both parents lived past 75—add 2 years. Neither parent lived past 75—subtract 2 years.
> 3. ***Exercise:*** More than 1 hour a day—add 2 years. More than 20 minutes a day—add 1 year. Less than 10 minutes a day—subtract 1 year. None—subtract 3 years.
> 4. ***Smoking:*** Never smoked—add 3 years. Quit at least 3 years ago—add 1 year. Smoke 1 pack a day—subtract 2 years. Smoke 2 packs a day—subtract 3 years.
> 5. ***Fiber in Diet:*** Five servings a day of fruits and vegetables—add 2 years. No fruits and vegetables in diet—subtract 1 year.

followed by the two ventricles beating in tandem. This electrical conduction system receives its oxygen primarily from the right coronary artery. If that artery becomes clogged with cholesterol plaques and can't carry enough blood and oxygen, the electrical system may become compromised, and bad heart rhythms may result. The most important of these is *atrial fibrillation,* the rapid vibration of the atria many times faster than the ventricles, resulting in an irregular heart rate and the loss of the "priming of the pump" by the atria, which in turn means a loss of about 25

6. ***Marital Status:*** Happily married—add 2 years. Married but with serious conflicts—add 1 year. Divorced—subtract 1 year. Single—subtract 3 years.

7. ***Blood Pressure:*** Between 90/50 and 120/80—add 3 years. Between 121/81 and 130/85—add 1 year. Between 131/86 and 140/90—subtract 1 year. Between 141/91 and 150/95—subtract 2 years. Above 151/96—subtract 3 years. (Note: Those who need blood pressure medications to achieve the above figures should subtract another year.)

8. ***Cholesterol:*** Less than 160—add 1 year. 200 to 240—subtract 1 year. 241 to 280—subtract 2 years. Above 280—subtract 3 years.

9. ***Body Mass Index:*** BMI of 19 to 22—add two years. BMI of 25 to 29—subtract 1 year. BMI of 30 to 31—subtract 2 years. BMI above 31—subtract 3 years. (A BMI below 19 is probably helpful, but in American society it is most frequently correlated with pathologic states such as anorexia, bulimia, hyperthyroid, or cancer.) (See Table 2.1)

※

percent of the heart's pumping power. The other two bad heart rhythms, caused primarily by poor blood and oxygen supply to the sinoatrial node, are *atrial flutter,* in which the atria usually beat three or four times faster than the ventricles, and *sick sinus syndrome,* in which the sinoatrial node continues to function, although erratically. Of the three, artrial fibrillation is the most common.

The other main causes of bad heart rhythms are heart attacks that damage the conduction system and congestive heart failure. The stretching of the heart muscle in congestive heart failure compromises the conduction system, predisposing the heart to bad rhythms. One of the main risk factors for this disease is uncontrolled high blood pressure; it is amazing how interrelated the various components and functions of the vascular system are.

In a heart attack, one of the coronary arteries has become completely blocked by a clot or a spasm of the artery, causing the heart to lose its blood and oxygen supply. Unless the artery is rapidly reopened with clot-busting drugs or *angioplasty* (elongated "balloons" that are threaded through groin arteries into the coronary arteries and then inflated), a part of the heart muscle dies and in time becomes a scar that no longer contributes to the pumping action, again predisposing the patient to congestive heart failure. If the heart's electrical conduction system is interrupted by a heart attack—usually caused by a blockage of the right coronary artery or the left descending coronary artery, which supplies it with blood and oxygen—the heart may suddenly stop beating and the patient may suddenly die.

These risks can be lessened through regular exercise, which keeps the coronary arteries open and develops collateral (or overlapping) circulation among these arteries—if one becomes blocked, the small offshoots of another take over and help supply blood and oxygen to the heart muscle and, equally importantly, to its conduction system. This helps prevent life-threatening bad heart rhythms such as *ventricular fibrillation,* which, unlike the similar-sounding atrial fibrillation, will result in death within minutes if not stopped with electrical paddles by your emergency room doctor.

Angina (chest pain) is caused by the narrowing of these coronary arteries so that, during exercise or under stress, the heart is no longer getting enough blood and oxygen. Although the result is temporary chest pain, seldom is there long-term damage. Angina is often managed in this country with "bypasses," in which one or more of the coronary arteries is replaced with a graft, usually from the saphenous vein in the leg or the internal mammary artery in the chest. Bypass operations are risky, often resulting in complications both in the heart and from strokes caused by clots produced during the operation. The bypasses rarely last more than ten years and would almost never be necessary if patients followed the kind of basic health advice I am going to talk about in this book.

Strokes, or "brain attacks," are most often caused by blockages in the *brain's* arteries. Significantly, the same kinds of clot-busting drugs that we have been using to treat heart attacks have now also been approved for treating strokes, so people who think they might be having a stroke should get to an emergency room as quickly as possible. Not only are strokes and heart attacks caused by the same process—vascular disease—but they are intricately linked in another way. When patients with heart disease develop atrial fibrillation, clots can form in the heart and travel to the brain causing an *embolic* stroke, a significant minority of all strokes. The most common of the three types of strokes is a *thrombotic* stroke, in which a clot originates in the brain itself. In a small minority of cases, strokes are *hemorrhagic* in nature, meaning that the wall of one of the brain's arteries has ruptured and bled.

SIDEBAR 2.3

New Drug to Lower Cholesterol

Most of us, fortunately, will never need to use a cholesterol-lowering medication, and those who follow the advice in this book are the least likely to need one. For those who are unable to control their cholesterol with diet and exercise, however, the decision of when to start medications is a tough one. There is abundant evidence that cholesterol levels are directly related to the risk of heart attacks. But the cardiovascular system is so central to our health that heart attacks are only one part of the story. Cholesterol-clogged arteries are also responsible for strokes, aneurysms, digestion problems, sexual dysfunction, and so forth.

Much of what we know about cholesterol and heart attacks comes from the Framingham Study, in which about one-tenth of the population of Framingham, Massachusetts has been studied since 1948 to determine almost every possible risk factor they might have and their health outcomes.

Three factors any physician must consider in deciding when to recommend starting a cholesterol-lowering medication, other than the obvious one of the patient's cholesterol level, are the side effects, the patient's willingness to lower cholesterol through diet and exercise, and the patient's age. The last factor is important because the relationship between cholesterol levels and heart attacks is less strong in the elderly. The field is fraught with controversy on this subject, and there is much room for legitimate disagreement among physicians. As a result, many patients with moderately high cholesterol go untreated, or are urged to modify their diet and to exercise, but fail to do so.

There are new data demonstrating that lowering cholesterol levels decreases the risk of heart attacks even in those patients who started at the high end of the normal range. I believe this strongly suggests that we physicians should be more aggressive that we have been about lowering cholesterol.

The most commonly used medications for this purpose are the *statins,* which do an excellent job and are almost always considered the first-line drugs for very high cholesterol levels. However, one of the oldest drugs for lowering cholesterol is the naturally occurring niacin, also known as nicotinic acid or vitamin B_3. (Despite its name, it has no relation to the nicotine in cigarettes.) This inexpensive and readily available vitamin, when given in large doses, is one of the most powerful cholesterol-lowering drugs available.

The limiting factor in the use of niacin has always been the skin flushing and itching that many patients experience when using it in the high doses needed to lower cholesterol. These side effects have been frustrating to physicians, because niacin is otherwise a powerful drug with minimal side effects.

In 1997, however, the FDA approved Slo-Niacin, an extended-release form of niacin. This preparation does not always eliminate skin flushing, but most patients find that they can be quite comfortable with its use, especially if the dosage is increased gradually. It is therefore ideal for patients with borderline high cholesterol, or as a second drug along with a statin for patients with very high cholesterol. Among the known side effects of both the older form of niacin and the slow-release form, other than the skin flushing and itching, are liver damage, higher blood sugars, and increased blood uric acid levels, which predisposes to gout. Fortunately, these side effects are rare and almost always disappear once the medication is discontinued.

Slo-Niacin is not a replacement for the first-line statins, but it is a welcome addition to the medical armamentarium for lowering cholesterol.

Hemorrhagic strokes most commonly occur in the *circle of Willis* (see Plate 4). This fascinating anatomical structure, first described by Dr. Thomas Willis in the seventeenth century, is a true circle of arteries that takes its inflow of blood from the two internal carotid arteries and the two vertebral arteries. The arteries flowing out of the circle supply the brain and the eyes with their blood and oxygen.

Several other types of vascular disease deserve mention (see Plate 4 for an overview of various vascular diseases). *Aortic aneurysms*—balloonings of the aorta most commonly found in the chest or the abdomen—can rupture, usually causing rapid death unless the patient is immediately transported to a hospital, diagnosed, and rushed to a surgeon waiting in the operating room.

In the broadest sense, *pulmonary emboli*—clots in the lungs—are a type of vascular disease. The clots usually start in the calves or the thighs and migrate via the veins to the lungs, where they cause potentially fatal blockages. Pulmonary emboli result from the same risk factors as the other types of cardiovascular disease, but physical inactivity and obesity predominate.

Mesenteric vascular insufficiency is a condition in which poor circulation in the arteries leading to the intestines can produce poor digestion or even pain in the abdomen when eating. It can progress to mesenteric infarction, or death of the affected portion of the intestines, a usually fatal outcome.

Peripheral vascular disease, usually referring to poor circulation to the feet, is rarely a killer, but only because most patients who have it die first of heart attacks. However, it causes severe impairment and, in the extreme, amputations.

One of the main risk factors for vascular disease is *hypertension,* or high blood pressure. The constant pounding of that pressure against the walls of the arteries causes arteries and walls to harden from fibrous deposits and thickening of the arterial muscle wall, and it predisposes them to the collection of cholesterol plaques, a type of *atherosclerosis* (see Plate 1). This *result* of high blood pressure, however, is also a *cause* of high blood pressure. The sensing of the blood pressure that allows the body to regulate it occurs in the kidneys. If the arteries to the kidneys—the renal arteries—are compromised by vascular disease, the kidneys sense the blood pressure as being lower than it really is, and they send a signal to raise the pressure, a condition known as *renal artery vascular disease.*

Thus, not only does high blood pressure cause vascular disease, but vascular disease causes high blood pressure—a classic vicious circle. The bottom line in all this is that, when the vascular system fails, hardly anything else works right either.

The various types of vascular disease are *all* caused by the same risk factors: smoking, a sedentary lifestyle, a high-fat diet, high blood pressure, obesity, and diabetes. Five of these six risk factors are within our control, and diabetes, while not curable, is manageable. Diabetes has a profound effect on the cardiovascular system, but I will scarcely touch on it in this book, because it is a book-length subject all by itself.

Table 2.1 Body Mass Index (BMI)

Height (ft, in.)	4,10	5,0	5,2	5,4	5,6	5,8	5,10	6,0	6,2	6,4	6,6
Weight (lb.)											
100	21	20	18	17	16	15	14	14	13	12	12
105	22	21	19	18	17	16	15	14	13	13	12
110	23	21	20	19	18	17	16	15	14	13	13
115	24	22	21	20	19	17	16	16	15	14	13
120	25	23	22	21	19	18	17	16	15	15	14
125	26	24	23	21	20	19	18	17	16	15	14
130	27	25	24	22	21	20	19	18	17	16	15
135	28	26	25	23	22	21	19	18	17	16	16
140	29	27	26	24	23	21	20	19	18	17	16
145	30	28	27	25	23	22	21	20	19	18	17
150	31	29	27	26	24	23	22	20	19	18	17
155	32	30	28	27	25	24	22	21	20	19	18
160	33	31	29	27	26	24	23	22	21	19	18
165	34	32	30	28	27	25	24	22	21	20	19
170	36	33	31	29	27	26	24	23	22	21	20
175	37	34	32	30	28	27	25	24	22	21	20
180	38	35	33	31	29	27	26	24	23	22	21
185	39	36	34	32	30	28	27	25	24	23	21
190	40	37	35	33	31	29	27	26	24	23	22
195	41	38	36	33	31	30	28	26	25	24	23

What Are Your Risks?

Height (ft, in.)	4,10	5,0	5,2	5,4	5,6	5,8	5,10	6,0	6,2	6,4	6,6
Weight (lb.)											
200	42	39	37	34	32	30	29	27	26	24	23
205	43	40	37	35	33	31	29	28	26	25	24
210	44	41	38	36	34	32	30	28	27	26	24
215	45	42	39	37	35	33	31	29	28	26	25
220	46	43	40	38	36	33	32	30	28	27	25
225	47	44	41	39	36	34	32	31	29	27	26
230	48	45	42	39	37	35	33	31	30	28	27
235	49	46	43	40	38	36	34	32	30	29	27
240	50	47	44	41	39	36	34	33	31	29	28
245	51	48	45	42	40	37	35	33	31	30	28
250	52	49	46	43	40	38	36	34	32	30	29
255	53	50	47	44	41	39	37	35	33	31	29
260	54	51	48	45	42	40	37	35	33	32	30
265	55	52	48	45	43	40	38	36	34	32	31
270	56	53	49	46	44	41	39	37	35	33	31
275	57	54	50	47	44	42	39	37	35	33	32

Table 2.1 Body mass index (BMI) is a rough measure of your health and life expectancy. The ideal range is about 19–22. The lightly shaded area (25–29) indicates overweight, a moderate threat to your health and longevity; the darker area (30+) indicates obesity, a serious threat. To calculate BMI on your own, divide your weight in pounds by the square of your height in inches, and multiply the result by 703. In metric units, divide your weight in kilograms by the square of your height in meters.

There is strong evidence showing that, with simple lifestyle changes, we could reduce the incidence of vascular disease to less than one-fifth of its current level. *We could thereby drastically reduce the cause of roughly 45 percent of all deaths and long-term disability in this country.* There is also strong evidence now that vascular disease is not just preventable, but even reversible. As one of the fathers of modern internal medicine, Sir William Osler, said, "Longevity is a vascular question."

Cancer

Cancer is a very different disease than vascular disease, but it turns out that many of the interventions that decrease the risk of vascular disease also decrease the risk of cancer. Cancer is the uncontrolled multiplication of human cells that should be reproducing at a controlled rate. Almost half of all cancers in the United States are caused by smoking, and many cancers are far more prevalent in those who eat a high-fat diet. The fiber in an ideal diet that helps to reduce cholesterol levels and prevent vascular disease also helps to prevent colon cancer. Exercise also reduces the risk of some types of cancer. A report by the Harvard School of Public Health released in November 1996 concluded that *nearly 70 percent of cancer deaths in the United States are due to poor diet, sedentary lifestyle, and smoking.* (I will discuss various forms of cancer, and how to prevent them, in later chapters.)

Thus, we can make dramatic reductions in the risk of the Big Three illnesses that cause 75 percent of all deaths in the United

States: heart attack, stroke, and cancer. And, as we have seen, the Big Three are really just the Big Two: vascular disease and cancer. We really do have far more control over the illnesses that cause so much disability and death than we once thought.

The *really* good news is that, in truth, controlling these risk factors doesn't mean sacrifice. For most of us, it does mean some profound lifestyle changes, but with a big-time payoff in the here and now. What I'm going to demonstrate to you in the rest of this book is that a lifestyle that controls these risk factors will also mean a greater sense of well-being, improved physical fitness, a more attractive appearance, a better sex life, fewer physical symptoms of illness, an improved ability to handle stress, and more intimacy and satisfaction in your relationships. Once you are on the pathway to superb health, you'll never want to go back.

What I'm also going to demonstrate to you is that the human body and spirit are so inextricably linked that it is difficult at times to say where the one begins and the other leaves off. I'm going to start by talking about how some very simple lifestyle changes will dramatically reduce your risks of heart attack, stroke, and even cancer. In time, though, you'll see that our inner lives—our sense of purpose, our sense of oneness with the universe and with others—dramatically affect our bodies' manifestations of health.

CHAPTER THREE

The Unified Field Theory of Health ❧

Recall a time when you raced home from school and your dog leaped against the fence, thumping his tail in excitement to see you. You grabbed your bicycle, a water bottle, and an apple, and pedaled off to the levee, the wind in your hair, as your dog cantered along beside you with his tongue hanging out and a doggie smile on his face, and all your cares dropped by the wayside.

Remember a time when you and your best friends clambered off the yellow school bus on the field trip, and you all raced up the trail together to the mountain brook and sat on the boulders. You pulled from your daypacks the tomato sandwiches and fresh nectarines your mothers had packed for you and washed them down with the sparkling, cold water streaming past your bare feet.

Think back to a time when all the kids were playing soccer. With the sun dipping below the hills and the stars beginning to come out, you kicked the ball and connected as you never had before. As the ball sailed into the net and the other players rushed to hug you, you knew you'd take on the world and never lose.

Some things about health are astoundingly simple. Attaining optimal health may be a process not so much of finding something we never actually had as of getting back in touch with things that were once second nature—of letting out that irrepressible inner child and that athletic, risk-taking inner adolescent.

Perhaps the biggest part of that journey back in time is the reawakening of the vigorous physical exercise we once took for granted and the healthful diet we once ate (until junk food became the norm)—interventions that are simple and seemingly trivial, yet absolutely essential.

Just as Einstein sought to develop a unified field theory of physics, there really is a "unified field theory of health." The five essential factors in a healthy lifestyle are diet, exercise, a strong social support system, freedom from addiction (especially smoking), and regular meditation. We will examine all of the five in this book, but for now we will concentrate on the two that dominate most people's thinking on the subject: the twin mantras of diet and exercise.

It's hard to find anyone who seriously disagrees that diet and exercise are beneficial to good health, but many people don't understand *how* they are beneficial, and I'm not at all sure that most people fully appreciate the extraordinary benefits they confer on us. When these benefits *are* truly appreciated, especially by those of us who are in second adulthood and prone to going downhill if we don't take care of ourselves, it's a lot easier to develop the self-discipline and make the lifestyle changes that are necessary to stay fit.

Exercise

Stronger and stronger evidence has accumulated, even in the last few years, that exercise is one of the absolute keys to remaining physiologically young and defying your chronological age. It is now very clear that exercise can in some ways actually *turn back* that physiological clock. There is new evidence, for example, that exercise improves memory and is protective against Alzheimer's disease.

Exercise opens up the coronary arteries, decreasing the risk of heart attacks, as well as develops "collateral" overlapping coronary arteries, so that the heart attacks that do occur will be less damaging. Exercise decreases blood cholesterol and blood pressure and helps maintain ideal weight, all of which dramatically decrease the risk of heart attacks. Regular exercisers have only about half the risk of heart attacks of nonexercisers, and those heart attacks that do occur in exercisers tend to be less severe because of collateral circulation, so the patients bounce back faster. Congestive heart failure is rare among exercisers. The greatest benefits are for highly trained athletes—heart attacks are a rarity in marathoners, whatever their age—but the really surprising part is how a little exercise will produce a dramatic benefit. Simply exercising twenty minutes three times a week to an exercise level that produces 80 percent of maximum heart rate will result in almost half the reduction of heart attack risk that the marathoner running fifty miles a week will enjoy.

Exercise decreases the risk of certain cancers, most notably breast cancer. It decreases the risk of diabetes, partly by helping to maintain ideal weight. But even independent of maintaining ideal weight, exercise helps to keep blood sugar levels normalized. And exercise dramatically reduces the risk of *osteoporosis,* the thinning of the bones due to loss of calcium that is particularly problematic for women after menopause.

Regular exercise can also dramatically improve your sex life. In men, exercise has been shown to increase both testosterone and human growth hormone levels. In women, it increases estrogen levels. For men, maintaining erections depends on keeping the penile artery open; regular exercise helps to keep cholesterol plaques from building up in that crucial artery, in the same way that it keeps the coronary arteries open (see Plate 5). In women, exercise helps to keep the pelvic muscles firm, making sex more pleasurable and less discomforting and making orgasms more intense.

Finally, exercise is a natural antidepressant and stress reducer. Regular exercisers suffer *far* less from depression and have a far greater sense of well-being than nonexercisers, and when things go wrong, exercisers feel far less stressed. This may be due in part to those famous *endorphins* (naturally occurring pain-relieving substances) that exercise releases and that simply make people feel good. The postexercise sense of well-being makes regular exercise a habit you won't want to give up once you've begun it. Couch potatoes have a real inertia about exercising, and there's no doubt that, for people who are not regular exercisers, it takes an investment to get started. But those who are regular exercisers feel so good when they exercise that they can scarcely imagine *not* exercising! For them, it's not a sacrifice at all, but a pleasure.

In the recent past, the prevailing wisdom in the medical profession was that the most important exercise was cardiovascular, and that the most important issue was to reduce the risk of heart disease. Cardiovascular exercise is no less important than it was, but more and more we're learning that weight training is also extremely important. Pumping iron dramatically decreases the risk of osteoporosis, which afflicts not just postmenopausal women, but many men as well. In men, weight training increases testosterone levels more than does aerobic exercise. And it improves physical appearance and self-esteem. There is new evidence that weight training is of great benefit even to the very old, including those in nursing homes.

One of the keys to developing a regular exercise program is choosing something you *like* doing. That may seem obvious, yet it's amazing how many people who hate running, for example, will start off their exercise program by doing just that. Despite their best

STAY YOUNG, START NOW

SIDEBAR 3.1

Exercise Self-Assessment

Finding the time and the self-discipline to exercise regularly is tough, especially with all of our modern conveniences that make it so easy to be sedentary. See how you rate.

1. On the way home to my condo on the third floor, I
   a. take the stairs, unless I'm carrying a bag of groceries.
   b. walk briskly up the stairs.
   c. take the elevator.
2. I get to work by
   a. walking to and from the train station.
   b. riding my mountain bike.
   c. feeling sporty and athletic while driving my four-wheel-drive sport-utility vehicle.
3. I make sure each muscle group in my body gets a workout by
   a. going ballroom dancing every week.
   b. exercising all muscle groups at the gym.
   c. playing cards, with special attention to wrist-muscle definition while reaching for the bridge mix.
4. I get regular aerobic exercise by
   a. playing golf.
   b. running five miles a day.
   c. surfing sports shows on Saturday TV, while being sure not to stop breathing.
5. My maximum heart rate is
   a. 70% of maximum on the stair-step machine.
   b. 80% of maximum while cross-country skiing.
   c. 60% of maximum while watching "code blue" scenes on the *ER* show on TV.
6. I recently joined a health club and planned to work out every day, but this week I'm too busy to go. I
   a. realize that my initial expectations were too high and decide to try going three times a week.

b. get a friend to join, and make plans to work out together every day.
   c. figure I've blown my health regimen anyway, so I might as well pig out on junk food.
7. I have an important report due at work tomorrow, and it's already late at night. I
   a. resolve to double up on exercise the next day.
   b. go to the local 24-hour health club and do the reading for the report on the exercise bike.
   c. stay up and do the report, staying awake by eating Skittles.
8. When I really don't feel like exercising, I
   a. exercise less vigorously than usual—for example, a moderate walk.
   b. motivate myself to stick with the program by focusing on the runner's postexercise "high."
   c. resolve to get back on the program just as soon as the stress in my life is over.

Scoring

Give yourself 3 points for each "b" answer, 2 points for each "a" answer, and 1 point for each "c" answer.

20–24 points: Superb! You are undoubtedly reaping the benefits of regular exercise: great appearance, unshakable sense of well-being, good sex, good health, and longevity.

16–19 points: Better than the average American, for sure, but there's still room for improvement.

11–15 points: You're average compared with most Americans—but in truth, that's not very good.

10 points or less: Couch potatoes of the world, unite—you have nothing to lose but your beer bellies.

intentions, they soon drop it out of boredom and frustration. Pick a sport you really enjoy. I personally don't much care for running, and if it were the only sport available, I'd never get enough aerobic exercise. But I can't get enough of ice hockey, and I totally lose myself in the adrenaline rush of the competition and get a really good workout every time.

Make exercising part of your social life. There's nothing more fun than a swimming pool party, a good pickup game of basketball, or a soccer game among friends.

If you're just getting started exercising, there's a lot to be said for a personal trainer to provide motivation and set up a regular schedule. Trainers aren't cheap, but many health clubs offer training services at affordable rates, and if that's what it takes to get you over the hump, go for it. The fast-paced aerobics workouts and high-energy music at most health spas these days will get almost anyone enthusiastic about exercise. And health clubs can be centers of social activity, with many offering health bars that are great places to meet people, as well as offering fitness weekends and outings that are sure to enhance your social life.

Consider whether you can make exercise a part of your commute. Many people these days bicycle, walk, or even jog to work. During my medical school days in the New England countryside, cross-country skiing was a popular way to get to school during the winter. And if your "commute" includes an elevator, take the stairs every day instead.

Once you're at work or school, try to make exercise a part of your daily routine. Some Fortune 500 companies even offer organized aerobics during the lunch hour, because they find it gets their employees' energy levels up for the afternoon.

For those who have physical limitations that preclude most conventional types of exercise, consulting a physical therapist is an extremely worthwhile investment. People who are unable to jog or play tennis may still find that they can stay active on a stationary bicycle or through water aerobics, and most communities these days have programs that can make this type of alternative exercise a part of your social life.

Finally, it's vital to be regular about your exercise. Make it a habit; if you lapse, it's all too easy not to go back. For those of us who are workaholics, this can be a challenge. If you really get stuck for time, don't forget that you can be doing your reading on a treadmill or stationary bike, so there's always time for at least basic exercise. And don't forget you can do calisthenics or jog in place in front of the TV set.

Exercise is best in moderation. The main benefits of exercise are in the leap from a totally sedentary lifestyle to a moderate level of aerobic exercise. While it's probably true that even greater levels of exercise will result in less heart disease and greater longevity, this "trained athlete" level of exercise comes at a price—the joint problems, fatigue, and increased free-radical production can actually result in faster aging. (For a discussion of what free radicals are and how they affect you, see the sidebar "The Antioxidant Revolution" in Chapter 12.)

Diet

The key to a healthful diet is to eat low-fat, low-cholesterol foods with a high fiber content, meaning lots of fruits and vegetables. This type of diet will dramatically reduce the risk of the various vascular diseases that cause more than half the deaths in this country, as well as improving men's sex lives by keeping the penile artery in good working order so that erections will come more easily. The low-fat, low-cholesterol component of this diet keeps the arteries open, reduces the risk of gallstones, and dramatically reduces the risk of various types of cancer—especially colon cancer, but possibly also breast cancer. The high-fiber component also reduces the risk of heart attacks. It does this in part by lowering cholesterol, since bile salts that are released into the intestines are high in cholesterol and tend to exit the body via the stool at a far higher rate with a high-fiber diet.

Also, high fiber may blunt blood sugar increases after a meal—increases that have long been observed to attack the walls of the arteries observed in studies on diabetics. A recent study showed that men who ate a high-fiber diet had only about two-thirds the rate of heart attacks as men eating a low-fiber diet, even after controlling for risk factors such as exercise and smoking.

One of the associations of family practice physicians, in fact, is promoting an "Oatmeal Challenge" for patients with high cholesterol. It has been shown that eating high-fiber oatmeal for breakfast every morning will lower cholesterol levels by about 10 percent in only one month. The "challenge," apparently, is to eat oatmeal every morning for a month without fail!

Fiber may also reduce the risk of colon cancer, a disease that is almost unknown in some primitive societies that eat a low-fat, high-fiber diet. Colon cancer hasn't received the same sort of public attention as other cancers, but it is the third most common cause of fatal cancers in both men and women, behind lung and prostate cancer in men and lung and breast cancer in women. The exact mechanism by which fiber may reduce colon cancer isn't completely clear, but it is known that digested food traverses the intestines faster in those who eat a high-fiber diet, thus decreasing their exposure to the carcinogens (cancer-causing substances) in the food they eat; the bulkiness of a high-fiber diet also reduces the concentration of carcinogens.

Fiber dramatically reduces the risk of another disease of modern society—*diverticulosis,* the little "outpouchings" on the side of the large intestine that can become infected (this infection is known as *diverticulitis*). These outpouchings are caused by the high pressures inside the intestines that result when food bulk is low, and they are almost nonexistent in those primitive societies that eat a high-fiber diet. In fact, diverticulosis was almost unknown in the United States until about fifty years ago, when we started eating white bread and other foods low in fiber and changing to a fast-food diet, which has almost no fiber in it. As one wag has commented, "Big stools, small hospitals; small stools, big hospitals."

With the kind of diet we're talking about, ideal weight can usually be maintained with little attention to total food intake. We now know that the calories in fat are far more dangerous to our waistlines than the same number of calories in proteins or carbohydrates. The risk of diabetes is much reduced by a low-fat diet, not only by helping to maintain ideal weight, but also by reducing blood sugar levels *independent of* weight. And a high-fiber diet will produce a feeling of fullness sooner than the same number of calories in a low-fiber diet, so the temptation to eat too much is reduced.

In our fast-paced society, it takes some care to avoid a fast-food (i.e., junk-food) diet. We're constantly bombarded with temptations—at the supermarket checkout stand, at the gas station, even on break at work when our "thoughtful" boss has provided us with doughnuts. It might help to remind yourself that with a low-fat, low-cholesterol diet, it's much less necessary to limit total food intake. You can go overboard on the three-bean salad or the whole-grain vegetarian sandwich with minimal guilt, whereas the bag of candy you pick up at the checkout counter will put a few ounces of fat on your hips or belly that it will take a while to get rid of.

It's true that the biggest offenders in the high-fat, high-cholesterol group are the red meats, beef, lamb, and pork, but chicken and turkey have received better press than they deserve. Chicken has roughly two-thirds the fat and cholesterol per unit weight of the red meats, so if you're serious, you need to cut back on chicken as well as red meat. In terms of its cardiovascular benefits, fish is without question better than any meat as a protein source, because the cold-water fish such as salmon and tuna contain omega-3 fatty acids, which actually seem to *reduce* coronary artery cholesterol plaques via a mechanism independent of overall cholesterol levels (more on this in Chapter 12).

Aside from the risk to your coronary arteries of a high-fat diet, it is the most important factor in obesity. Americans have become fatter year by year, even after adjusting for age; in other words, it's not just the aging of the population that is producing more overweight people, but the constant temptations of our junk-food culture.

Obesity is the enemy of longevity and optimal health. Those who are significantly over ideal weight are at greater risk for diabetes, high blood pressure, and many other maladies. Molière hit the mark when he observed, "The fork has killed many more than the sword."

Following a low-fat, high-complex carbohydrate diet (meaning wheat bread, oatmeal, etc.) will leave you feeling better simply by making it easier to maintain ideal weight. Perhaps more importantly, though, it will "smooth you out" emotionally by releasing sugar into the bloodstream more slowly, in contrast to the emotional liability and "sugar blues" caused by a junk-food diet. And there is new evidence that a high-complex carbohydrate diet will decrease the incidence and intensity of migraine headaches.

What is so remarkable is how interrelated all of these health inputs are. If you've tried to change just a few of these practices, it was probably hard, because it was hard to notice a difference. If you're willing to go for the whole program, the supportive feedback

SIDEBAR 3.2

Getting Started

One of the toughest parts of a makeover is getting started, overcoming the inertia that has kept you from being in shape in the first place. Especially if you are significantly overweight, as many Americans are, it can be tough to visualize yourself feeling fit and energetic.

The first thing to remember is to enlist the support of others. If you sign up for a health club or get involved in a sports team, the examples of other people just like you who are accomplishing what they want will keep you going. Again, enlist a friend or do it with a partner.

One of the best exercises for getting started (in fact, one of the best exercises, period) is simply brisk walking. You can increase your distance a little each day, and no one ever said you can't stop for a rest if you need one.

For those who have been used to a typical American diet, a low-fat diet can seem like deprivation at first. Remember, though, that diet is an acquired taste. Once you have been drinking nonfat milk for a while, whole milk starts to taste like cream.

Stay on the program, and in time the positive feedback from your body about all the right things you're doing will keep you on track.

your body will give you will be so overwhelmingly positive that it will be hard to turn back.

Notice in Figure 3.1 how complex the interrelationships are. This diagram is actually very simplified, yet for most people without medical training, the cause and effect at each point in the diagram will take some thought and study to understand. I'm describing only three factors in this diagram—diet, exercise, and smoking—yet even those three result in an extraordinary complexity of correlation. Imagine the further complexity if I added even one extra input: the damaging effects of poorly managed emotional stress or of social isolation. The resulting interrelationships would take a three-dimensional chart to depict!

I've already noted that fear of death isn't really much of a motivator, so let's turn the diagram around. Instead of depicting all the *damage* done by a sedentary lifestyle, a poor diet, and smoking, let's look at the *benefits* in the here and now from regular exercise, a good diet, and the other three factors in the Big Five, as depicted in Figure 3.2.

This time, resolve to go for the paradigm shift, the fundamental lifestyle changes that will allow you to punch through inertia and give you the payoff you're looking for: the greater energy, the sexier look, the self-esteem, and the profound sense of well-being that go with the program.

For those who have been sedentary and out of shape for too long, it's sometimes difficult to remember what it was like to be active and fit. When you're tempted to skip your workout at the

STAY YOUNG, START NOW

Health Consequences of a Sedentary Lifestyle, Poor Diet, and Smoking

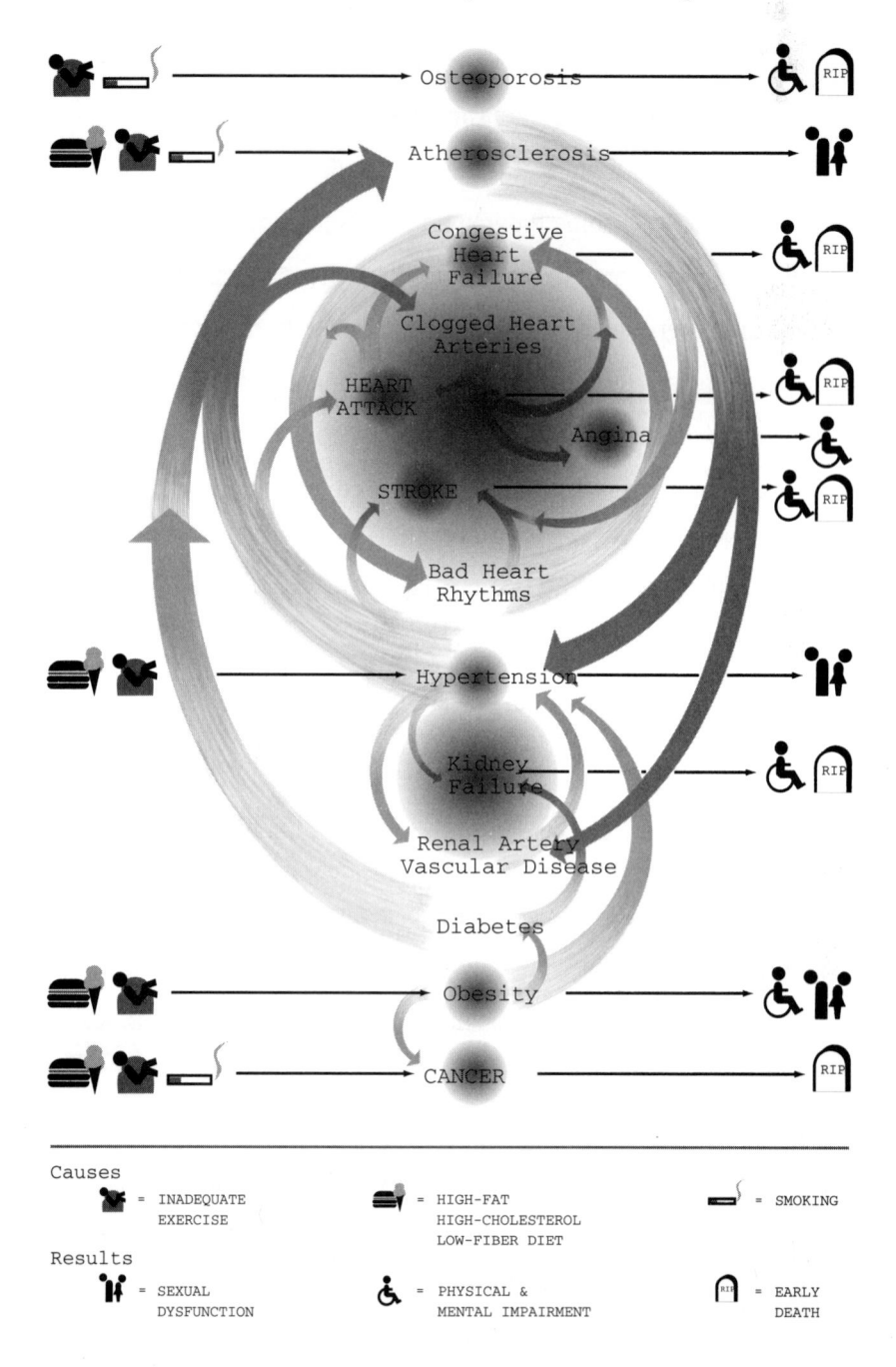

- Osteoporosis
- Atherosclerosis
- Congestive Heart Failure
- Clogged Heart Arteries
- HEART ATTACK
- Angina
- STROKE
- Bad Heart Rhythms
- Hypertension
- Kidney Failure
- Renal Artery Vascular Disease
- Diabetes
- Obesity
- CANCER

Causes
- = INADEQUATE EXERCISE
- = HIGH-FAT HIGH-CHOLESTEROL LOW-FIBER DIET
- = SMOKING

Results
- = SEXUAL DYSFUNCTION
- = PHYSICAL & MENTAL IMPAIRMENT
- = EARLY DEATH

50

The Unified Field Theory of Health

Benefits of the "Big Five" Lifestyle Cho

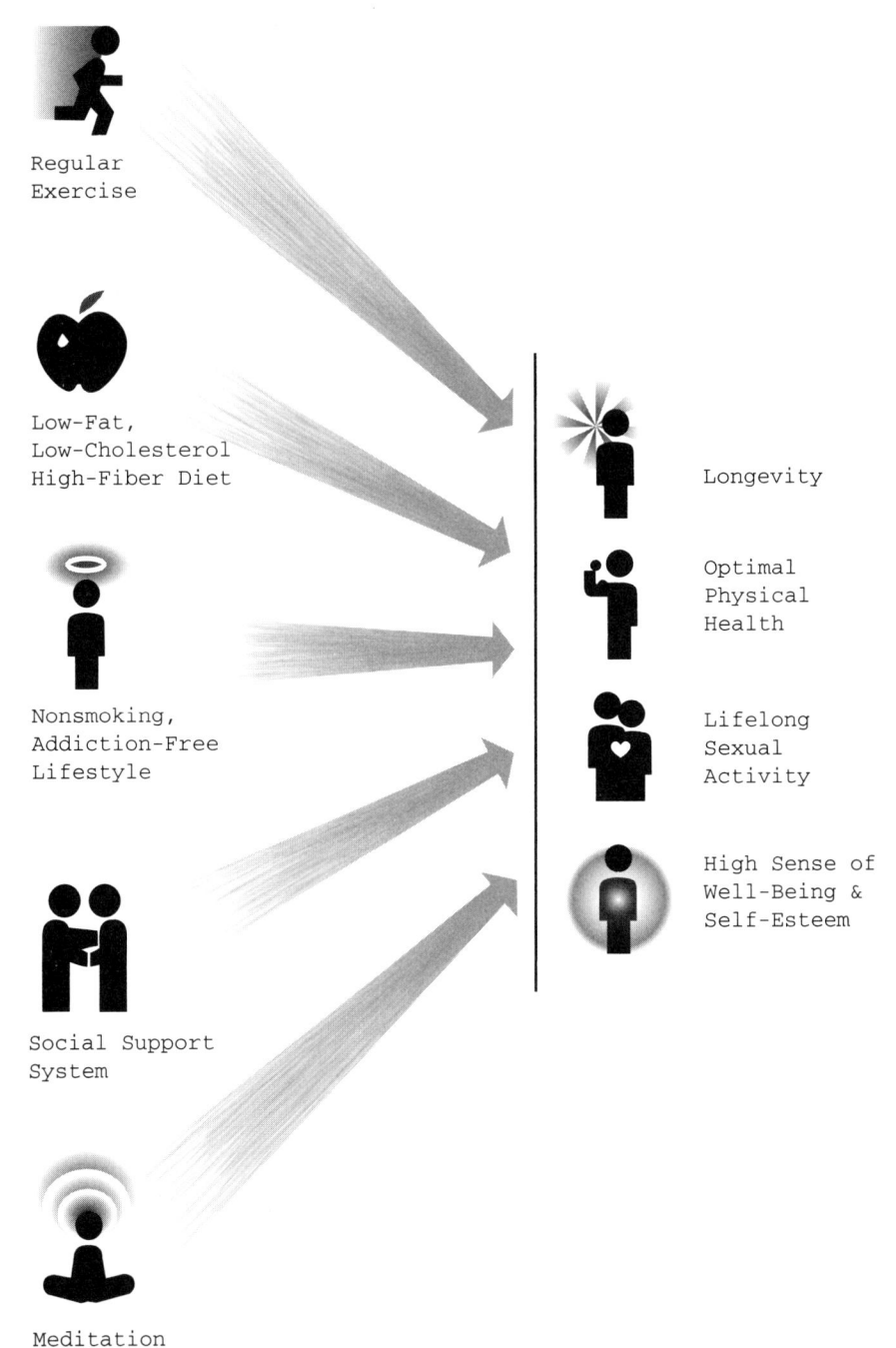

Regular Exercise

Low-Fat, Low-Cholesterol High-Fiber Diet

Nonsmoking, Addiction-Free Lifestyle

Social Support System

Meditation

Longevity

Optimal Physical Health

Lifelong Sexual Activity

High Sense of Well-Being & Self-Esteem

health club, though, or you're hit with the urge to make a pit stop at the drivethrough fast-food joint, recall for a moment those carefree days not so many years ago when you felt such simple joy with your friends out on the playing field. That inner adolescent is still there, and that youthful body is still waiting to reemerge if you give it the chance. Stick with the program, and the day will come when taking care of yourself is second nature. The powerful sense of well-being you'll experience will keep you from ever turning back.

CHAPTER FOUR

The Mind/Mind Connection ⚜

The existence of the mind/body connection is almost a cliché, and it is difficult even to watch a TV talk show without seeing some manifestation of that awareness. I am more and more convinced, however, that the mind/body connection is just the tip of the iceberg—that the real story is the mind/mind connection, the ambivalences and contradictions we feel that lead us unwittingly to send the body a "mixed message" reflecting our unresolved subconscious conflicts.

The mind/mind connection that we will explore later in this chapter in no way detracts from what we have learned about the mind/body connection—knowledge that is now real and commonplace to almost all of us. Almost everyone can think of a friend or relative who, although deathly ill, desperately wanted to see a certain milestone in his or her life and just made it before dying. I vividly remember a young nursing student in my premedical physics class whose dying grandmother desperately wanted to see her granddaughter graduate from college. This tenacious lady held on just long enough to be able to walk unaided to the graduation, only to die a few days later. The drama was made all the more compelling because her granddaughter had an aversion to physics and passed the course by the skin of her teeth—unbeknownst to her grandmother.

I remember that, as a beginning medical student, before I had gotten out onto the wards, I had the mental image of cancer patients doing everything they could to survive, of asking for specialist after specialist and requesting one experimental treatment after another. I imagined them reacting as though they'd been exhorted by Dylan Thomas with his immortal lines, "Do not go gentle into that good night. / Rage, rage against the dying of the light."

Many patients *are* like that, of course, but there are far more who are generally accepting of their fate and who find their diagnosis of a terminal illness almost a respite from the disappointments that life has dealt them. Dr. Bernie Siegel, in *Love, Medicine and Miracles,* noted the same phenomenon—that when he began his Exceptional Cancer Patients group, only a tiny fraction of the patients he invited showed up for the free seminars. It's certainly not hard to see how the reactions of fatalistic patients to their prognosis will hasten their demise. But neither is it hard to understand how the unfailing will to live and to succeed would keep alive the great physicist Stephen Hawking, who has cheated death for years despite the usually grim prognosis of his amyotrophic lateral sclerosis (Lou Gehrig's disease), or how Mario Lemieux could bounce back from life-threatening leukemia to become the National Hockey League's Most Valuable Player, or how Lance Armstrong could recover from testicular cancer and go on to an amazing win in the 1999 Tour de France bicycle race.

The effect of one's emotional state on one's body can be documented scientifically. For example, a study done in 1996 at the Mayo Clinic showed that after angioplasty, the coronary arteries of patients who were generally very hostile and who easily became angry closed up two and one-half times faster than those of patients who were not hostile. Another striking study, released by the Johns Hopkins School of Public Health, also in 1996, showed that depression increased a person's risk of heart attack fourfold, even after controlling for risk factors such as smoking and high blood pressure.

Various studies have been done of how many people seeing a physician in a general practice clinic have a mind/body issue, or in medical jargon, are "somaticizers"—people whose bodily complaints reflect the stress in their lives. The numbers I've seen have ranged from 25 percent to 60 percent, but they underestimate the problem, because almost all of the remaining patients who have organic illness have psychological reactions produced by the illness itself: anger, denial, depression, assuming the "sick role," etc.

The mind/body connection has been known to medical science at least since the second-century Greek physician Galen noted that melancholy patients got cancer more often than those who had a

SIDEBAR 4.1

Heart Attack Risk Self-Assessment

Research is increasingly showing that a key risk factor for heart attacks, independent of diet, sedentary lifestyle, smoking, and so forth, is negative emotions and how we handle them. Feelings of anger, cynicism, anxiety, and hopelessness can predispose to heart disease. See how you rate in managing your emotions.

1. I still haven't set aside nearly enough money for my retirement. When I confront my financial future, I
   a. think it will work out, but I still spend some sleepless nights worrying about it.
   b. feel less anxious after I've taken some concrete steps, such as enrolling in financial planning courses.
   c. think, what future? The Indians and Pakistanis have the bomb, a worldwide depression is just around the corner, and global warming will submerge my home.

2. When I'm invited to help out with my local youth group, I
   a. ask them to call back next year, when I expect to be less busy.
   b. recall the "helper's high" and the great people I met the last time I volunteered, and say "yes."
   c. don't let myself get sucked in.

3. I'm in a long line at a tollbooth. The toll taker gets flustered, and people begin honking. I
   a. say nothing, but glare at her as I give her the money.
   b. smile and commiserate with her about the stressful day she's having.
   c. tell her in no uncertain terms that she'd better find another job if she can't count change.

4. My spouse does something that disappoints me. I
   a. point out that this is yet another example of how he or she doesn't meet my standards.

b. express my frustration in terms of how I feel when he or she acts that way.
c. give my spouse what he or she deserves: the silent treatment.

5. I'm at a community meeting called to protest the development of a uranium mine next to my subdivision. I
   a. look around for somebody I know already.
   b. feel a little nervous that there are so many unfamiliar faces, but introduce myself to the first friendly looking person I see.
   c. go home after having a glass of punch. I don't know anybody, and besides, nobody cares what I think.

6. After my yearly physical, my doctor tells me my cholesterol is high. I
   a. lash out at my spouse for suggesting that I give up some of my favorite high-fat foods.
   b. go for a walk with my spouse and the family dog, and talk over how to confront this challenge.
   c. wish my spouse hadn't talked me into the checkup. What's the use—heart attacks run in the family.

7. I finish painting the garage Sunday afternoon. I
   a. chide myself when I notice that the second can of trim paint was a slightly different shade than the first.
   b. celebrate by throwing a party for the friends who helped me work on the job.
   c. work myself into a fit as I realize that, with the lousy quality of paint these days, I'll have to redo it in three or four years.

8. I discover that a famous television evangelist used some of the proceeds from his charity appeal for an expensive weekend with his secretary. I
   a. write to the TV network, expressing my indignation.
   b. remind myself of my good fortune that some of my own indiscretions have never appeared on nationwide TV.

c. am not surprised. I've long since learned to distrust people who are always soliciting donations.
9. After years of hard work, I'm passed over for a promotion in favor of someone nobody knows from the man in the moon. I
   a. am inwardly angry, but do my best to outshine that person.
   b. decide it's past time to start my own business.
   c. start plotting ways to make the new-hire look bad.

Scoring

Give yourself 2 points for each "a" answer, 3 points for each "b" answer, and 1 point for each "c" answer.

24–27 points: Excellent—you're a good example of "attitude is everything."

20–24 points: Very good—you're succeeding most of the time in staying in a constructive frame of mind.

15–19 points: Careful—your sometimes negative attitude may be more of a risk factor to your health than your blood pressure or your cholesterol.

9–14 points: Hmm—perhaps the Ghost of Christmas Future really *does* have a message for you.

※

greater sense of well-being. Unfortunately, it remains a mystery to many contemporary physicians.

Physicians, and especially medical school professors, pride themselves on a scientific approach to medicine, and rightly so. But that scientific approach is often taken to such extremes that it becomes a disservice to the medical community and to patients. For example, there is overwhelming evidence of the health benefits of a strong social support system, of the healing power of touch, of regular meditation, and of spiritual life and a sense of meaning and purpose in patients' lives. Nevertheless, these crucial influences on our health seem to be off the radar scope of all too many physicians, perhaps because they weren't discovered in a chemistry or biology laboratory.

Even psychiatrists, traditionally the most people-oriented of all physicians, sometimes fall into the trap of pill pushing at the expense of talking with their patients. There is no question that a huge amount of mental illness is due to biochemical imbalances, and we are fortunate to have new and far more powerful generations of antidepressants and antipsychotics. But the availability of these new drugs has led some physicians down the path of neglecting to talk with their patients and address their emotional and spiritual issues. What we are left with is a medical profession that sometimes seems irrationally rational and illogically logical.

The result is that patients and their physicians often speak two different languages. I have seen interactions in which the patient is describing a physical symptom such as a headache, how it first occurred at a friend's funeral, how it worsens when the children misbehave, and how it occurs at certain times of the day or after eating certain foods. The physician, however, often plays the role of the rational scientist, asking if this or that pain medication has been tried or whether a CT scan of the brain has been done. Sometimes, in these *deux solitudes* discussions, it seems that the patient has more insight than the physician into the true source of the problem.

All too many physicians, when confronted with patients who are somaticizing, inwardly label their stories "crocks," and may even tell them, "There's nothing wrong with you; it's all in your head." Yet the body so often *is* a reflection of our problems that it can serve as a marker for the stresses, the difficult choices, and the evasions in our lives. It is the wise physician who can help patients explore, in a safe environment, what is really going on in this regard. That ability distinguishes the true healer from the mere technician.

A patient of mine named Sandra once complained to me about chronic back and shoulder pain that had started about three weeks earlier. Her X rays were negative, and, in any event, for someone only in her early forties and in otherwise excellent health, she was at low risk for a compression or hairline fracture. When I explored with her what was going on in her life, she related that she had become the caretaker for her much older husband, who was suffering from ankylosing spondylitis, a debilitating, arthritislike condition that was keeping him bedridden most of the time. Although Sandra tried to put the best face on things, she was, in fact, a vibrant, young-at-heart woman who would have much preferred to be riding her mountain bike or scuba diving rather than taking care of an invalid, a duty that seemed to stretch far into the future. As we discussed her situation, she suddenly blurted out, "You know, Doctor, I sometimes feel that the pain in my back and shoulders is symbolic, like I'm carrying my husband. What do you think?" And, of course, she was right.

The Mind/Mind Connection

I did my basic family practice training on the Navajo Indian reservation in Arizona. As a medical student, what brought home to me the reality of the mind/body connection was the stark realization that the illnesses it causes are culture related. Hardly a day went by in my clinic in which a Navajo patient didn't complain to me about a band of pain circling around the waist all the way to the back. In the years since, I've *never* heard such a pattern of pain described among my Anglo patients—but I've seen plenty of pain in parts of the body where pain is unknown to the Navajo!

Perhaps more telling, however, is the radically different way the Navajo would deal with such illnesses. A traditional Navajo medicine man would spend from half a day to three full days with a sick patient. The history that would be taken would include the whole story of the patient's family, as far back as could be remembered, including any curses placed on the family and what each family member had died of. The patient's illness would be chronicled in minute detail, including each symptom and precisely how the patient felt at that time. Finally, the medicine man would perform a ceremony and attempt to exorcise the demons that had caused the illness.

If we were to analyze the medicine man's history of the family and early life of the patient in modern medical terms, it could be seen as dealing with unresolved family conflicts, with the patient's childhood problems, and with his or her extended family and social support system. The curses on the family could represent the recurring issues the patient perceived as unavoidable. The chronicle of the illness itself is a concept as old as Freud's "talking cure" and as new as some of the principles behind the science of neurolinguistic programming. The truth is that, for the many bodily problems that have their origin in the mind/body connection, the Navajo medicine man often has more to offer than modern medical science.

In the early 1990s, two studies showed a strong correlation between irritable bowel syndrome and childhood sexual abuse. Irritable bowel syndrome is a classification of chronic bowel problems that do not seem to have any organic cause: diarrhea, constipation, or pain with defecation, with all diagnostic studies negative. It is found mostly in women, which is, I believe, because of women's tendencies to turn emotional issues inward and to somaticize or become depressed. Men, by contrast, are more likely to lash outward and to hot-rod, kick the dog, or blast away at beer cans with a hunting rifle when they are frustrated or angry. Since women are far more likely to have been sexually abused in childhood, the connection between sexual abuse and irritable bowel syndrome was intuitively plausible.

After learning of these studies, each time I had a female patient with irritable bowel syndrome I would tell her, in the most non-threatening way I could, "There are some new studies showing that there is a correlation between irritable bowel syndrome and childhood sexual abuse," then ask, "Could this possibly apply in your case?"

Of the twelve women I asked, *nine* told me that, yes, they had been sexually abused in childhood or adolescence. My own group of patients didn't constitute any kind of scientific study, but the experience brought to me in a flash—in one of those great "Aha's" that life sometimes offers us—that for these women, the illness was a manifestation not just of the sexual abuse they'd undergone, but of their *inability to communicate it.*

Children and adolescents who were sexually abused were invariably threatened by their abusers and warned not to talk to others about it. Even later in life, when their abusers were long gone, the women were faced with the dilemma that even in our more open, modern society, some issues are difficult to discuss, and a stigma is still attached to having been victimized. Therefore, they had had no alternative but to unconsciously turn their anguish inward and suffer in silence.

My sense of what was going on proved accurate in time. When I encouraged the women to open up, either with me or with a supportive psychotherapist, about what was going on within themselves, most—although not all—reported improvements in their irritable bowel syndrome brought on by this emotional release. What worked for them—at least, for most of them—was to describe to a caring and supportive professional precisely what had happened in the abuse and precisely how this had affected their lives, and to describe precisely their bodily symptoms, with each word chipping away, little by little, at the hold the past had on their present health.

The mind/body connection will come as little surprise to most, but what complicates it infinitely is that, in truth, we are often of more than one mind. I'll never forget a patient I knew from medical school, Beth, who had undergone a radical form of brain surgery. The brain is divided into the left hemisphere, which controls the right half of the body, and the right hemisphere, which controls the left half of the body. The two hemispheres are connected primarily via a bundle of nerves known as the *corpus callosum*. As a last resort in epileptics for whom no known drug combination has controlled their seizures, the corpus callosum is sometimes surgically cut, leaving the two sides of the brain with hardly any neural connection. This prevents seizures from propagating throughout the entire brain, but it also prevents the two hemispheres from communicating (a syndrome that is also found in people congenitally lacking a corpus callosum—a rare disorder. Since (in right handed people) the left side of the brain is responsible for rational thought and the right side is the more emotional, more expressive and artistic side, at times Beth was literally "of two minds."

"Sometimes my left hand—the more impulsive hand—reaches out at the dinner table for a dessert, but the rational right hand knows it isn't good for me, so it reaches out and pulls the left hand back," Beth told me. "Last week I was talking on the phone about a business deal with a colleague I don't like very well. I knew I had to put up with him, but I made the mistake of holding the phone in my left hand. When he said something rude to me, my left hand slammed down the phone. It's a real problem sometimes, but at least it's better than having seizures and waking up on the floor not knowing who or where I am."

Gregory currently sees me for his schizophrenia. Gregory is a junior college student whose wire-rimmed glasses give him an intellectual appearance, and in fact he is gifted both in mathematics, excelling in his calculus courses, and as a jazz pianist. Like most schizophrenics I have known, he is a heavy smoker.

Gregory does well most of the time, but if he forgets to take his Prolixin—an antipsychotic in the same class as Haldol or Thorazine—he hears voices in his head that torment him with derision and urge him to kill himself. Most of the time, Gregory is an insightful young man, but when the voices become too persistent and too loud, he sometimes asks me, "Doctor, are those voices real?" On occasion the question has struck me as an existential one—for Gregory, the voices are real enough.

Another patient of mine from medical school—without question the most memorable patient I've ever had—suffered from multiple personality disorder. MPD is found in people—almost invariably women—who have been terribly sexually or physically abused as children. Having no way to resist, they pretend that the abuse is happening to someone else. Eventually this depersonalization takes on a life of its own, and the patient develops multiple personalities, some of whom have no memories in common with one each other.

In truth, a good many patients who describe themselves as having MPD don't have the problem at all and are just mimicking what they've seen on TV. MPD is a real enough psychiatric diagnosis, however, and no health professional who knew Vicky, my patient, doubted that her MPD was genuine.

Although each MPD patient is unique, typically there will be a primary personality that is mild-mannered and meek, as the Vicky I knew was. The second most frequently seen personality will typically be an angry one, enraged and bitter about how she has been treated. The third personality is often a seductive one who can express the sexuality not permitted by the main personality.

Vicky had all three of these personas—and several others, including even a young girl. By the time she was my patient on a mental hospital ward, she had begun, after years of intensive psychotherapy, to integrate her personalities into a whole. After six weeks on the ward, I had seen only her main personality, the mild and meek Vicky I had come to know. I'll never forget, however, the sudden appearance of her secondary, angry personality.

I was chatting with Vicky when she began ruminating about a TV program she'd seen that day about child abuse. In mid-sentence, she leaped out of her chair and shouted at me, "And who the hell are you?" Her neck veins were engorged, and her mouth was twisted into a menacing snarl. This woman's face was different, her voice had changed, and her body language was threatening in a way that was out of character for the Vicky I had grown accustomed to. I had read about how the various personalities of MPD patients would have different blood pressures, warts and rashes that would change, and even color blindness in some personalities but not in others. However, nothing I had read had prepared me for this extraordinary transformation that seemed to have come straight out of a thriller movie. Eventually the Vicky I knew returned, apologetically explaining that she had "lost time." I was relieved, yet profoundly troubled by what I had seen.

Admittedly, these three patients represent extremes—Beth with her two sides of the brain that can't seem to agree, Gregory with the disembodied voices inhabiting his mind, and Vicky with her multiple personalities. And yet, I'm increasingly convinced that, in more subtle ways, all of us are frequently of more than one mind.

An everyday example of this principle is the often-observed fact that depressed patients rarely are successful in stopping smoking. While they may say that they understand the dangers of smoking and want to quit, in fact there is a suicidal component to depression that makes people want to behave in self-destructive ways. (To further complicate this example, in one of medicine's many vicious circles, some of the chemicals in the witch's brew of cigarettes *cause* depression.)

Another everyday example is that of patients who on a conscious level believe they would like to lose weight but are held back from it by an unconscious block. I have often seen female patients who seem to be doing everything right, yet who are substantially overweight and can't seem to bring their weight down. Sometimes when I've asked them how their husbands or boyfriends reacted when they began to lose weight, they have replied, "He gets very nervous, and starts to worry that I'll go out with other men." In that ambivalence is the answer to why weight loss is so difficult for them. (Interestingly enough, I've never seen such a response in men. I don't know why.)

In truth, we are all a jumble of contradictions, some of them existing only on unconscious levels. All of us "adults," if we search hard enough, will find not only an inner child but also an inner adolescent, and we men have our feminine side, just as women have their masculine side. Most of us are happy to be alive, yet I have never met a patient who, on close questioning, didn't acknowledge having contemplated suicide at some time.

That, obviously, complicates enormously the mind/body connection. Even those patients with the strongest will to be healthy and live a long and happy life have a part of them that is content to be sick, to take time out and be taken care of. And even those people who will unhesitatingly tell you they want to die have, in fact, a part of them that wants very much to live. This is why fewer than one suicide attempt in five is "successful," an oxymoron if there ever was one and a phenomenon with which, as an emergency physician, I am intimately familiar.

Many of us go through life blissfully unaware of our ambivalences and our inner contradictions, but they are there if we look hard enough. We can maximize our chances of getting what we want in life if we know what it is and focus on attaining that goal. When we *don't* get what we want—when life gives us the booby prize—it is most often because there was a part of ourselves that was ambivalent: an emotional, and sometimes unconscious, side of us that was heading in another direction entirely. If we can identify that ambivalence, identify the payoff that part of us got by holding back, that insight will help us to align ourselves to succeed. By no means does this call for being self-judgmental, but simply for looking within and seeing what's so for us.

It has become almost trite to observe that resistance to illness is reduced in people who are stressed or depressed, but the real story is far more complex than that. In truth, there can be one part of our psyche that is vibrant and purposeful, while another part is slogging along, happy to undermine our good health. Even the most cocky and confident among us approach life's goals with that small inner voice telling us we won't succeed; that inner voice is only too happy to send us flu symptoms or a migraine headache that will give us the excuse not even to try.

Many have observed that the more sociable among us enjoy better health than do the introverts. Part of this is simply the intimacy with others that is so universally cherished and so crucial to our well-being. Another part is that the world is a mirror to us, and it is in communicating with others on a deep level that we get a glimpse of our own ambivalences, of the multiple sides of our personalities. It is in looking at those ambivalences that we can put them in order and get the "Aha's" in life that reveal to us why we feel the way we do.

In the previous chapter I talked about keeping the body's plumbing in order, and I do hope that it inspired you to go for the fruits and veggies and work up a sweat at the gym. Here I want to add one of the absolutely key components to radiant good health, and that is *communication.*

As you walk the road of life, share who you are. Share your innermost self, and listen to what your fellow travelers on that road are sharing about themselves. I promise you, not only will the imperfections in your body that hold you back become less troubling, but as you share with those closest to you, as each mixed feeling, each indecipherable emotion is explored, what you will find deep inside is the gift of self-awareness and insight, and the miracle of self-acceptance.

CHAPTER FIVE

No Man Is an Island &

The poet John Donne once said, "No man is an island, entire of itself." The struggle between belonging and alienation, between connectedness and drift, between meaning and emptiness, is a central feature of our lives and is of crucial importance to our well-being and our physical health.

- In a study of almost seven thousand men and women living in Alameda County, north of San Francisco, those who were socially isolated had a two- to threefold increased risk of death from heart disease *and* all other causes of death, independent of risk factors such as cholesterol level and blood pressure.
- A study at the University of South Florida demonstrated that older Japanese living in the United States who had preserved their traditional lifestyle had far less cognitive decline, such as Alzheimer's disease, than similarly aged Americans, whereas

ethnic Japanese in the U. S. who had adopted American ways showed no such advantage. After extensive surveys of diet and other factors that might explain this difference, the investigators concluded that it was the *human contact* that counted—that the Japanese tradition of welcoming the elders in the home until they died kept them feeling involved and loved, and kept their minds occupied and their faculties sharp.

- At the Ohio State University College of Medicine, scientists found that patients who scored above average in loneliness had significantly poorer immune-system functioning and were thus more susceptible to disease.
- At the Medical College of Wisconsin, researchers found that unmarried persons with cancer had a decreased overall survival rate, even after adjusting for disease severity and type of treatment.
- In a study conducted in Michigan, 91 percent of serious complications during pregnancy occurred among women who had little social support.

The data confirming the crucial importance of our social support system are unequivocal and well described even in the traditional medical literature, yet most practice in our health care system goes against this knowledge of our social links. In obstetric wards, the family is often separated from the expectant mother, and the miracle of birth occurs in isolation. In emergency rooms (although not in mine, thank you), the patient's family and friends are sent to the

> **SIDEBAR 5.1**
>
> ## Internet Use and Depression
>
> In the fall of 1998, researchers at Carnegie Mellon University released a study showing that the more people used the Internet, the more depressed they became. The psychologists who conducted the study were surprised, as they had expected that the Internet would allow people to feel more connected with others who had similar interests.
>
> In truth, though, we are all social animals, and we need genuinely human contact rather than seeing words and images scroll across a computer screen. Physicians have noticed for hundreds of years that people who are shut-ins because of illness become depressed. Part of that depression, of course, is simply because they are sick, and part of it is because they are unable to exercise—the greatest and most natural cure for depression. However, a huge component of the depression of shut-ins is simply their lack of human contact.
>
> Human beings are hardwired to desire contact with others, and that interaction needs to be "face time," where we truly feel the presence of others and sense how *they* feel by the clues of their facial expressions, their body language, and their vocal inflections. The Internet has a place, just as does the television, that much older promoter of social isolation and sedentary lifestyle, but both have a feature that should be used more often: the switch that turns them off.

waiting room while the frightened patient awaits the unknown in a stressful environment among strangers. By contrast, in Third World countries, when a patient is hospitalized, the family virtually moves in as well, lovingly cooking the patient's food and helping to nurse

SIDEBAR 5.2

Americanization Can Be Bad for Your Health

A recently released study conducted by the University of California at Berkeley has shown that U.S.-born Mexican-Americans have *twice* the level of psychiatric disorders compared with Mexican-born Hispanics who immigrated to the United States or with Mexicans living in their homeland. The researchers found that, by the third generation of residency in the U.S., the rates of adolescent risk behavior—such as violence, drug abuse, and unprotected sex—approached or exceeded those of adolescents from American families of many generations.

The most important factors in the skyrocketing levels of psychiatric illnesses among the immigrants were the breakdown in the extended families that are the norm in Mexico, the lack of the socially enforced safe behavior in the villages from which most of them came, and the long working hours here that tend to isolate parents from their children.

Numerous other studies have shown that the higher-fat diet and decreased levels of exercise in the United States compared to Mexico have resulted in Mexican-Americans who have higher levels of obesity, higher blood pressure, and higher rates of diabetes than their counterparts who stayed in Mexico.

Most Americans are accustomed to thinking that we have the world's best health care, and it is undeniably true that Mexican-Americans live longer than Mexicans in Mexico. It is also true, however, that some of the most basic health-care interventions, such as a strong social support system, good diet, and regular exercise, are more common across the border in Mexico, a country we often think of as "developing." In our rush to be more modern, we may have left by the wayside a few customs and values that served us well in bygone times.

him or her back to health—yet another example of how our modern technology has taken us away from our roots.

These data are all the more crucial when we realize that in our modern society we have to make an effort to build and nurture our own community. Not so long ago, we lived in one town, walked to school, and later walked to work. We grew up with the same people, and the idea of community was something we took for granted and scarcely thought about.

Today, the Internet links us more than the town meeting, and millions of Americans are road warriors living out their lives in airports and Holiday Inns. It is still possible to create and nurture our own community, but it takes effort and resourcefulness, and millions who can't or won't make the effort are left isolated and alone. We now have overwhelming scientific evidence to support what we really knew all along: that those with well-developed social support systems stay healthier, live longer, and are just plain happier.

What we all want, ultimately, is to be loved and understood, to feel that someone or some people "get" who we are and what we are experiencing at the deepest levels. Whether it be our satisfaction in our achievements or simply our joy in watching a sunset, we want to share ourselves and what we are going through with people who care.

All of us have had disappointments in our lives that sometimes have left us feeling angry, sad, frustrated, unloved, or depressed. For those who withhold communication, these negative emotions persist. Those who, on the other hand, can tell the truth—both to themselves and to others—are physically and emotionally healthier. For example, if you can acknowledge, "I wanted a relationship, but in the frame of mind I was in at that time, I found myself looking for people who were wrong for me," you will find that not only is the negative charge removed from that issue, but it also opens up the space for the relationship you want. If you can say, "I wanted my business venture to succeed, but I found I wasn't tough enough in negotiations to make viable agreements," that telling of the truth—that saying it the way it really was—unravels the bitterness, sadness, and regret, and allows you to move on.

Telling the truth and sharing ourselves doesn't just mean sharing what has gone wrong for us, but also sharing the true miracles in our lives—our love for those close to us. How many of us have regretted not telling someone how much we cared about them, only to have them move away and lose touch, or even die unexpectedly?

In the Broadway play *Carousel*, the protagonist, Billy Bigelow, a fairground barker, is unable to tell his dear wife, Julie, of his love for her, and during his short life the closest he can come is to say, "If I loved you." When the dead Billy is permitted a single day to return to earth to his widow, who for fifteen long years has been a single mother, he sings to her:

If I loved you,
Time after time I would try to say,
All I want you to know . . .

Billy then finds within himself the strength to tell Julie what has always been locked in his heart: his deep love for her. In his last moments of his one day on earth, he holds her tightly in his arms and pours out to her how much she has always meant to him.

Carousel touches people so deeply that if the curtain were to fall and the lights come up too quickly, we'd see tears streaming down the faces of grown men. It touches all of us on a deep level because there isn't one of us who doesn't have regrets about waiting too long to say "I care."

Communication is crucial to our well-being, and I am convinced that much of the healing ability of the most accomplished healthcare professionals comes not just from their knowledge of medicine, but also from their willingness to listen attentively to their patients—to their pains and their sorrows, their triumphs and their tragedies. Everyone has heard of the placebo effect, the ability of a sugar pill dispensed by a physician to make a patient feel better. I believe a good part of the placebo effect is not simply that the patient believes in the healing qualities of the physician and the medicine, but that the communication of his or her ailments to a caring professional—simply describing them accurately to someone who truly understands what is said—helps the pain to diminish or disappear.

After my stint on the Navajo reservation, I did my family practice residency at the Jewish General Hospital in Montreal. During my psychiatry training there, my supervising psychiatrist asked me if I wanted to help lead a support group for Jewish

SIDEBAR 5.3

Social Support System Self-Assessment

With so many Americans spending increasing time on the road in ever more complex and stressful jobs, our social support system and sense of community that we once took for granted can now prove to be elusive, and keeping that sense of family and community intact takes work. See how you rate.

1. When I come home and find things in disarray, I become irritated at the sloppy maid service in my hotel—until I suddenly realize that I'm not *in* a hotel:
   a. Sometimes.
   b. Never.
   c. I'm never home.

2. I have a hard time remembering the names of my children's friends:
   a. Sometimes.
   b. Never.
   c. Are you kidding? The tough part is remembering *my* children's names.

3. The most profound conversations I've had recently with my spouse and children were
   a. on the telephone.
   b. while relaxing together on our recent family vacation.
   c. via e-mail.

4. I met my oldest friend
   a. in college.
   b. in elementary school.
   c. at a business meeting for my current employer.

5. The associate I know best by first name is
   a. my boss's administrative assistant.
   b. my child's teacher.
   c. the concierge at the Chicago Hilton.

6. I feel most comfortable discussing my most intimate feelings with
   a. the therapist I often consult via telephone from my hotel.
   b. my spouse or significant other.
   c. sorry, I don't divulge my intimate feelings.
7. Lately I've been spending most of my free time
   a. making repairs around the house.
   b. enjoying life with my spouse and kids.
   c. planning our company's downsizing.
8. I volunteer time with people in an organization that is dear to my heart:
   a. Once in a while.
   b. On a regular basis.
   c. Are you kidding? I don't even have time to be a "volunteer" for my family.
9. My spouse and I
   a. work different shifts.
   b. work the same shift.
   c. both hold two jobs.
10. I'm offered a higher-paying job in a faraway city where we have no family or friends.
    a. I persuade my spouse and children to join me in the new city.
    b. After talking things over, my spouse and I decide that our family, friends, church, and children's school are more important than the money.
    c. I move to the new city, and stay in touch with my spouse and children by phone during the week and with weekend visits.

Scoring

Give yourself 3 points for each "b" answer, 2 points for each "a" answer, and 1 point for each "c" answer.

> ***26–30 points:*** Congratulations! You have managed to keep your family and community life working in a world in which it isn't easy.
>
> ***21–26 points:*** Like most of us, you need to concentrate a little harder on this crucial area of your life.
>
> ***16–21 points:*** No question that this aspect of your life needs attention.
>
> ***15 points or less:*** A real road warrior. Better keep your photo on the mantle so your family will recognize you when you come home.

concentration camp survivors, who make up a surprisingly large percentage of Montreal's aging Jewish population.

My first reaction was, "Good grief, here I am in one of the most cosmopolitan and exciting cities in the world, and this guy wants me to devote my free evenings, without pay, from my already frantic schedule, to help people who have gone through something I'll never be able to understand—and I'm not even Jewish!" So my initial reply to him was a flat no.

Within a few days, though, the idea had grown on me. More and more, I realized that these were people who could teach me more than I could teach them, and I concluded that the experience of going into the lion's den with patients who had gone through pain, suffering, and loss beyond what I could imagine would help to prepare me for whatever might happen in my work as a physician.

Several of the participants, as it turned out, were patients of mine from the Herzl Clinic at Jewish General, all of whom had charts as thick as encyclopedias, filled with exhaustive studies of their migraines, their chest pains, their abdominal pains, and their insomnia. They were people who had never had the chance to mourn, and who, immediately after their liberation from the camps, had boarded ships for Canada and had gotten on with making a living and restarting families with other survivors.

When I think back on my five months with them, tears come to my eyes. My social worker colleague and I encouraged them to talk and talk, and we taught them meditation techniques that, for more than one, unlocked happy prewar memories.

Can you imagine their most bitter complaint—these people who had lost all family, all friends, and all material possessions? *That they had not been believed about what had happened!* Their attempts to communicate their loss to the world had often been thwarted by the unwillingness of the world to accept what they were saying, by the disbelief of many people that such a holocaust could actually have occurred. As tough as it was sometimes, my colleague and I listened and listened and listened, in many cases to elderly people in the twilight of their lives.

And on the last day, after we had held a ceremony to light a candle for the fallen, they told us what the group had meant to them. They were sleeping better. Their headaches and abdominal pains had gotten better. And their relationships with their children and grandchildren had been transformed. I hadn't touched my stethoscope or reached for a prescription pad, yet the transformation in the health of these patients had been beyond anything I had seen the most advanced technology produce. For month after month, they had slowly assuaged the grief of their terrible losses, word by word releasing the grip in which the past had held them.

As Albert Camus said, *"Crushing truths perish from being acknowledged."*

CHAPTER SIX

The Healing Power of Touch ✖

One of the most riveting dramas in all of medicine is the struggle for survival in the neonatal intensive care unit. In windowless rooms under harsh fluorescent lights, tiny premature babies weighing no more than two or three pounds fight for a toehold on life, under the watchful eyes of masked and gowned nurses. The "preemies" thrash fitfully under the Plexiglas windows of Isolette incubators, their tiny cries barely audible through the plastic walls surrounding them.

In a remarkable demonstration of the healing power of touch, it has been shown that preemies who are massaged for fifteen minutes three times a day are far more likely to win their fight for life. They gain weight almost 50 percent faster. They sleep better. They leave the hospital sooner. The simple act of being comforted by a warm, caring hand seems to do more for them than all the tubes and monitors and warning bells that surround them during the drama of the weeks or even months of their tenuous grasp on life.

The healing power of touch has been known to medicine since at least the time of Hippocrates in the fourth century B.C., yet, over two millennia later, physicians often forget it. I'll always remember the time in my medical school training when I diagnosed an appendicitis in a patient on a psychiatric ward where I was doing a clerkship. I summoned the surgical team on call to get this poorly educated schizophrenic admitted to the surgical floor. The intern from the team arrived, and, after looking over the tests I had ordered and examining the patient, came to the same unavoidable diagnosis I had made. The patient, however, adamantly refused an operation.

What followed was a parade of physicians who perfectly describe the pecking order in academic medicine. The second on the scene was the first-year resident, who also could not persuade the patient to undergo the operation voluntarily and who mumbled about a "5150," medical-legal jargon for forcing a patient considered incapable of making rational decisions to be admitted against his will. Such a course involved the risks of the time loss inherent in going through the legal system, as well as the risk in trying to put a patient under anesthesia involuntarily.

The parade continued up the hierarchy: second-year resident, third-year resident, fourth-year resident, chief resident, and finally the senior attending surgeon. None was successful, and in fact the patient was digging in his heels more than ever.

The Healing Power of Touch

Finally the entire surgical team arrived en masse. While holding their conference outside the patient's room, the chief resident clutching the legal papers needed for an involuntary operation, the attending motioned the team medical student to have a go at trying to persuade the patient voluntarily. "You're the only one who hasn't talked to the guy," the attending said. "See if you have any luck."

The medical student had hardly been in the room two minutes when she came out with the news that the patient had changed his mind and agreed to an operation. My own attending, a psychiatrist who had watched in bemusement as the whole minidrama unfolded, suggested that we use the situation as a learning experience and see if we could deduce what had changed the patient's mind.

Each of the surgeons described all the logical arguments and warnings of death he had made to the patient. It turned out, though, on close questioning by the psychiatrist, that each had argued with the patient while standing across the room from him.

The medical student, not having had the "benefit" of all these bad examples, had shaken the patient's hand—the only one to do so, as it turned out—and then sat on the bed next to him, put her hand on his shoulder, and said simply, "We're very worried about you"—at which point the patient almost immediately agreed to the operation.

The "laying on of hands" has a healing power that was often all that physicians had in the days when medicine was more of an art than a science. Accomplished physicians will almost always listen to a patient's heart and lungs, however unlikely it may be that this exam will help in the diagnosis, because it is an excuse to place one reassuring hand on the patient's shoulder and the other hand over the heart, so often experienced as the seat of love, spirituality, and emotions.

One of the classic wars in medicine has been the never-ending battle between orthopedists and chiropractors, the former contending that chiropractic has no scientific basis. It is undeniably true that chiropractic cannot budge a slipped disk, nor can it restore, over the long term, a subluxed vertebral body (one that is improperly aligned). Yet many patients under chiropractic treatment get better—something that can't be said for many of my patients who have had back operations. There is undoubtedly a science to chiropractic, but I am convinced that part of chiropractic's benefits come simply from the human touch of a caring D.C.

There is increasing evidence that the power of touch—whether it be from a massage therapist, from physical therapy, or even from the physical linking with a close friend or family member—will help virtually any illness with a mind/body connection. Asthma, migraines, depression, and a legion of other ailments all respond to the warmth of human touch.

Americans may laugh at the French custom of kissing friends on each cheek, but the much greater physical closeness among family and friends in the French and many other Latin cultures has been shown to translate into much lower levels of violent behavior than we see in American society. When lovers meet in a French café, they will be seen to touch each other every few moments, while an American couple in a booth at the local Mel's Drive-in will usually be more verbal and less physical.

Many have observed that a dog or cat can do wonders for the sick, in particular for older shut-ins. Dogs especially offer us not just the unconditional love that is so often lacking in our human relationships, but the physical closeness and nuzzling that can often feel sexually threatening when coming from another person. It is a sad commentary that there is such an epidemic of sexual harassment or even abuse that many people, especially women, often feel threatened by physical closeness.

It is unlikely that the reserved American culture will change anytime soon to be more like the physically demonstrative Latin culture, but at least we can remember to make the effort to be physically close in our own families. Children need to have their hands held, to sit on the laps of their parents, and to be hugged often. Couples need to remind themselves to take the time for the physical closeness we need every day, and to reconnect at that most basic level of human interaction.

Perhaps one of the most striking and insightful studies about the healing power of touch to come out of the scientific laboratory was conducted by Dr. Janet Quinn, who measured an index of immune function in patients receiving therapeutic touch. She found that not only did immune function improve in those *receiving* therapeutic touch, but it improved just as much in those *giving* it. Quinn's study speaks to us in a way that most dry scientific studies cannot, because it gives us not only an insight into the biological mechanism of the healing power of touch, but also the beginning of a scientific confirmation of the healing prayer that St. Francis gave us centuries ago when he told us, "*It is in giving that we receive.*"

CHAPTER SEVEN

Sexual Fulfillment in Second Adulthood

Making love can be that most intense of human experiences, that deepest intimacy with another in which our shared sensuality takes us into another world and leaves us filled with warmth and tenderness—Shakespeare's "very ecstasy of love." That physical and emotional intimacy and understanding may well be the closest we come to total union with another, to the feeling that we are truly not alone.

On the other hand, there is so much survival tied up in sex, so much evolutionary angst about finding a sex partner and reproducing, that when things go less perfectly than in romance novels or on the big screen, the experience can be pretty anxiety provoking.

As we leave behind our adolescent and young adult lives, our style of making love changes gradually but dramatically. Speed and frequency of intercourse and sexual gymnastics tend to take a back seat, to be replaced by communication, tenderness, and intimacy, and our lovemaking slows down to take advantage of our deeper understanding of our partner's needs.

Many men beyond their thirties and forties find themselves losing interest in being the conquering, promiscuous male and begin to focus on intimacy and depth with a single partner. Such noted playboys as Warren Beatty can now be seen in monogamous relationships, cooing over their new babies, and even Hugh Hefner broke down and cried openly at his marriage, short-lived though it turned out to be. When Sylvester Stallone's first daughter was born with a defective heart and had to undergo surgery, the excruciating wait led to a profound transformation, and he took her survival as a gift from above and an omen. "You can go out and look for variety and novelty," he said, "but, c'mon, at the end of the day, who are you going to open your heart to, a sexual encounter or someone you've literally been to hell and back with? I've slain my last dragon. I'm a changed man."

Women in their thirties, forties, and beyond often find that they are better able to communicate their thoughts and emotions and are more able to be assertive—all acquired skills that lead to a greater ability to achieve intimacy. And the end of the childbearing years can often lead to more time and energy for a deepening relationship with the person they love.

The physiological changes we undergo can, however, leave us yearning for our younger bodies. For men there is usually a general decline in sex drive and, perhaps more importantly, a decline in the ability to achieve and maintain an erection.

Many women, on the other hand, experience an *increase* in libido with passing time. Both the Kinsey and the Masters and Johnson studies showed that, while men are generally at their sexual peak early, in fact in the midteen years, many women's interest in sex *grows* with time. It is sometimes not only greater postmenopausally, but the liberation from worries about unwanted pregnancy and the end of often uncomfortable menstrual periods can free women to be more open and uninhibited about an active and joyful sex life than ever before. Women's anxieties tend to revolve around their body image, their psychological and physiological changes following the menopause, and their new self-image following the conclusion of the years of fertility. Sometimes they have difficulties with a sexual partner who is not showing enough interest in sex to keep them satisfied, or even difficulty in finding an appropriate lover at all. On the other hand, many women do experience a decrease in libido postmenopausally.

Obviously, these are gross generalities. A minority of men, especially those who have always enjoyed an active and satisfying sex life, will find that they have barely slowed down in their forties. Some women, especially those whose love lives have been disappointing or who have had traumatic early-life experiences with sex, will welcome an end to sex altogether. Two other factors that can produce a decrease in libido for women are the changes in the years surrounding the menopause—although fortunately this usually lasts no more than two years—and a "surgical menopause," or hysterectomy, that is not accompanied by appropriate hormonal replacement therapy.

The *good* news is that for most of us, most of the time, sex only gets better. Previous generations had the preconception that enjoyment of sex stopped at a certain age, but all we need to do to dispel that myth is look around and see people of our age having the time of their lives. I have found, over and over, that the bumps in the road are often due to lack of understanding of the physiological changes that we all go through. In my practice, I have rarely found couples who were unable to profit enormously from a holistic approach to sex, with counseling, education, improved communication, and attention to some of the basic health issues that we've already discussed. What follows is what you need to know to make your second adulthood the most sexually satisfying years of your life.

Men's Issues
(Required Reading for Women)

Men may generally find their interest in sex gradually declining as they get older, but for most men the limiting factor is not interest but rather a slowdown in their ability to get erections. A big part of that problem would be solved by Viagra, but most men nat-

Sexual Fulfillment in Second Adulthood

> **SIDEBAR 7.1**
>
> ## Health Benefits of Regular Sex
>
> - Sex is a form of exercise. Couples who have sex three times a week burn off about 7,500 calories each in a year.
> - Regular sex increases testosterone levels in men and estrogen levels in women. This improves the overall hormonal milieu of both men and women, but it is especially important in women wishing to conceive.
> - Regular sex decreases cholesterol levels by a slight but measurable amount.
> - Regular sex results in better sleep, just as regular exercise does.
> - Regular sex almost certainly decreases the rate of prostate cancers.
> - Sex releases endorphins, just as aerobic exercise does. Those who suffer from chronic pain such as headaches or backaches will find the pain lessened if they can have regular sex. (Guys, take note: You now have a new comeback to the "I have a headache" excuse!)

urally would prefer to be able to have working erections without the need of a pill.

The process of getting an erection is actually a physiologically very complex interplay between the vascular system, the nervous system, the hormonal system, and the emotions. Let's discuss each of these in turn.

The Vascular System

The vascular system is by far the main factor as to why it becomes harder to get hard with time—it is the same old story of the plumbing I've discussed previously. The penis becomes erect by engorgement with blood, which is supplied by the penile artery. That artery, sadly, isn't very large—it's much smaller, in fact, than the coronary arteries that cause us so much grief when they get clogged up—and the reasons it goes downhill with time are exactly the same as the slippery slope of coronary artery dysfunction: a high-fat, high-cholesterol diet, a sedentary lifestyle, and smoking. The onset of that downhill slide varies enormously, but most men will notice a slowdown beginning in their thirties.

How fast the decline occurs depends largely on lifestyle choices, as well as the medical problems of poorly controlled blood pressure, high cholesterol, and diabetes. Of course, sex is a pretty powerful motivator to stick to the twin mantras of diet and exercise, and I've seen over and over again that men who were nonchalant about the risk of a heart attack *really* started to pay attention when I explained to them the links between their lifestyle and their ability to get an erection. I'll never forget a Hell's Angels patient of mine during my internship who couldn't care less about "going out with the big one," but who paid rapt attention to what it would take to keep his harem satisfied, and who gave up smoking to that end.

Nevertheless, even men who have paid careful attention to lifestyle issues will gradually see a change in their sexual response.

This is usually first noticed as a slowing down in erections while fantasizing or seeing an attractive woman. Men sometimes mistakenly label this "impotence," when in fact it happens normally with the passing of the years. If you have a difficult time achieving an erection with visual imagery, but you can become erect and ejaculate by masturbating or with stimulation by your sex partner, you are not impotent at all, but are simply going through a normal physiologic change that all men will experience sooner or later, even if they may not talk about it in the locker room.

Many men remain silent about these issues with their wives, their friends, and even their physicians. Those who do bring them up with their physicians often see the problem as a "lack of male hormones," and some come to me and say, "Doc, I need a shot of testosterone." I have only rarely gotten to the point of prescribing testosterone, because on close questioning, the problem almost always turns out to be not a lack of interest in sex, but rather a slowdown in erections. Testosterone is not only pretty peripheral to that problem, but also is a drug with its own set of side effects, the most serious of which is prostate enlargement, but also including salt and fluid retention and a worsening of diabetes. A much more intelligent way to increase testosterone levels is through regular exercise that increases muscle mass. I say intelligent because when testosterone levels are increased in this more natural way, rather than by injection, the body's internal control systems remain intact and functioning, and the higher levels of testosterone are much more likely to be beneficial and without side effects. Not to

> **SIDEBAR 7.2**
>
> ## Viagra for Erection Difficulties
>
> Viagra works! Viagra (sildenofil) has truly proved to be the breakthrough drug anticipated by physicians who do sexual function counseling, with a record number of prescriptions having been written during its first few years on the market. It is highly beneficial for most men with erectile dysfunction, but many other men who can achieve near-normal erections are experimenting with it for a sexual "edge."
>
> Taken about an hour before sex is anticipated, Viagra comes in tablets of 25, 50, and 100 milligrams. In the same class as the injectable Caverject that has been available for years, it works not only by opening the penile artery (and its branches) entering the penis, but also by temporarily closing the veins leaving the penis, thereby almost perfectly mimicking nature's signal for an erection. Because it also opens the genital arteries in women, it may prove also to be a boon to many women who have difficulties achieving orgasm, especially those with risk factors for atherosclerosis (which affects the genital arteries): postmenopausal age, smoking, sedentary lifestyle, high cholesterol level, and diabetes.

mention that exercise is cheaper than seeing your doctor and a lot more enjoyable, and provides a host of other benefits as well.

When men are worried about their ability to achieve an erection, it is all too easy simply to roll over in bed and feign disinterest. But the cost in loss of intimacy and sexual fulfillment is tremendous. And, since maintaining sexual function depends on being sexually active, just as staying fit demands a minimal level of exercise, forgoing sexual relations due to fear of erectile dysfunc-

> Side effects can include headaches, diarrhea, flushed skin, upset stomach, and vision distortions involving the color blue. In men the most potentially severe side effect is *priapism,* an erection that lasts more than four hours, which not only can be very painful but can also result in long-term erectile dysfunction. This risk is probably strongest for men who experiment with the drug in larger doses than recommended, but it can also be a problem for men with sickle-cell anemia, a blood disorder affecting blacks almost exclusively.
>
> Viagra should *never* be used simultaneously with nitroglycerin or any other nitrate drug, since all these drugs tend to lower the blood pressure, and the result can be life threatening.
>
> For all the success of Viagra for many men—and women—it should be remembered that the clinical success rate for the men taking it in the trials was 60 to 80 percent, meaning that a significant minority of men experienced little or no benefit. For those men, the other treatments discussed in this chapter remain an option. And for men *and* women, Viagra should not become an excuse to neglect the cardiovascular fitness that will make lifelong sexual function possible *without* the use of a pill.

tion risks entering a vicious circle in which sexual function goes further downhill.

What this underscores is the need for communication and mutual support in lovemaking. Men, you need to open up! If you sometimes put off having sex because of performance anxiety, you need to tell the truth. You need to say to your partner, "I sometimes put off having sex because I'm afraid I won't be able to get an erection." What do you have to lose? If you *don't* say what you're really feeling, you've just chucked overboard the intimacy and openness in your relationship—and what's left of any value if you don't have that?

And if you can take that first step, the next step of expressing what you need to make your sex life work will be that much easier. What most men in this situation need is direct stimulation of their penis by their partner, and if you can express that, and understand that you're far from alone in what you're going through, you're on your way.

Women, you need to be supportive! There is very little about a man's ego that is more fragile than his lovemaking abilities. It is crucial to having an active and satisfying love life to make your man feel wanted and sexy. Being judgmental isn't going to get you very far. Even if it's true that your man contributed to his problems by smoking, drinking, eating bacon and eggs, and being a couch potato, harping on this will never turn him into a better lover.

Women, it is important to realize that, even though you may have spent most of your life with men who were willing and able to perform whenever the opportunity presented itself, the tables are turned if you have a sex partner who is experiencing difficulties in achieving an erection. Especially if you are at a point in your life when your sex life is more important than ever, if you are in the mood for sex and he is worried about performance, *you* are now a threat to *him*.

One of the most important things you can do in this situation, after full and open communication, is to be a truly active participant in lovemaking and give your man a lot of direct stimulation of his penis. Although most women now in their teens and twenties feel free to be active and equal participants in sexual relations, there still seem to be a fair number of women from earlier generations who feel that it is up to the men to take the lead in lovemaking and that it is somehow less than feminine to be truly an equal partner sexually.

Talk things over, perhaps even with the help of a relationships counselor or sex therapist. If you are truly open with your partner, you might well find not only that whatever fears you may have of being perceived as unfeminine and whatever early childhood messages you have internalized about "how it is done" are *not* shared by your man, but that he will eagerly welcome any changes that would allow your sex life to really take off.

Talk over together what seems to work in maintaining erections, and how both of you feel about those possibilities. One fabulous option is oral sex, a choice some couples seem to resist. Oral sex can be extraordinarily satisfying, both to men and to women, and many men can maintain erections far better this way. Some people have concerns about the cleanliness of oral sex, but in fact it is no more "unclean" than deep kissing. Many couples enjoy the "69" position, in which the two partners give each other oral sex simultaneously. Others enjoy lovemaking in which they start with oral sex and then proceed to intercourse.

You might also consider different positions. Some men enjoy direct hand stimulation of their penis right up until the moment of

> **SIDEBAR 7.3**
>
> ## Two New Drugs for Erection Difficulties
>
> Following the blockbuster drug Viagra, there are two new oral drugs in the pipeline for erection difficulties. Vasomax (phentolamine) is an oral version of the injectable drug that has been in use for some time. Apomorphine (the generic name; there is no brand name yet) is used sublingually, meaning under the tongue. Both drugs may prove useful for those who have not benefited from Viagra. It will probably be possible to combine two or more of these drugs for optimal results.
>
> Both of the new drugs are expected to be available in U. S. pharmacies no later than mid-2000, and Vasomax is already available by prescription in Mexico.

penetrating of the vagina. Other men find that they can maintain erections more easily by making love "doggy style," and many women as well enjoy variety in lovemaking positions.

The Nervous System

The second factor in the ability to achieve an erection is the nervous system. Erection and ejaculation are an interplay of the two components of the *autonomic*—meaning involuntary—nervous system, namely the *sympathetic* system and the *parasympathetic* system. The parasympathetic system promotes relaxation and is essential to achieving an erection. The sympathetic system is the "fight or flight" side and is essential for ejaculation. Thus, for successful sexual performance, there has to be a balance between being relaxed and yet excited enough to perform.

The significance of this in the modern age is the effect of stress on sexual relations. Most of us need and thrive on at least a moderate amount of stress; that's what gives us the sense of life as a game, and without it we'd be bored. But too much stress—meaning a level at which we feel we can't keep up with what life is throwing at us, no matter how hard we try—is notoriously hard on sexual relations, especially the ability to achieve erections. A couple that is having sexual problems that seem stress related might do well to work out a common strategy to reduce the stress level, or at least to have some protected time and privacy as a couple.

The nerves in the autonomic system usually work well throughout our lifetimes, but there are three exceptions. Heavy drinking is the cause of one of them. Male alcoholics almost always have severe erection problems by the time they hit their forties, because drinking pickles those crucial nerves that control erections. Women with drinking problems will also notice a decrease in sexual responsiveness, especially in the ability to achieve orgasm. Going on the wagon improves performance dramatically, but it is rarely possible to turn back the clock completely to the pre-alcohol state. I get pretty upset about alcohol and cigarette commercials aimed at teenagers, touting these addictions as sexy; it's hard to think of things more *damaging* to a healthy sex life than booze and tobacco.

The second factor that can dramatically affect the nerves themselves is diabetes, which is a triple hit because it also attacks both the arteries and the veins. I've scarcely talked about this problem, because diabetes is a book-length subject all by itself and is beyond the scope of what I can cover here. Suffice to say that if you are diabetic, stick to the program your doctor advises, bare though it always is.

One last thing that can affect the nervous system and lead to erection problems is prostate surgery or radiation therapy. The nerves that control erections are tiny, and they pass so close to the prostate that, during surgery or irradiation, even in the best of hands, they can be damaged. Urologists are now more than ever aware of this problem, and many make a special effort to do microsurgery that spares the sexual nerves.

The Hormonal System

The third factor in achieving an erection is the hormonal system. The blood testosterone level tends to go down in men with the passing of time, but since it starts out at such a high level, it remains high enough for excellent sexual function for the lifetime of most men. When men have difficulty getting an erection as they get older, it is almost always more likely to arise from problems with the vascular system due to plaque deposits on the walls of the arteries than from low levels of testosterone. This can be confirmed with blood tests, and urologists have sophisticated methods of evaluating the blood flow to the penis.

A much simpler, and generally very accurate, way to determine the cause of the problem, however, is to ask yourself if you get sexually turned on and yet find that an erection does not always result. If this is the case, the problem is most likely vascular, especially if you have risk factors such as smoking, high blood pressure, or high cholesterol. A minority of men will be exceptions, and if blood tests confirm a low level of testosterone, then testosterone replacement might well have a big impact on their sex lives. These days, testosterone replacement is generally accomplished with a convenient skin patch.

The Emotions

The final factor in achieving an erection is the emotional dimension, and one of the biggest problems is depression, which decreases libido in both men and women. Depression is a very common issue, and one that I urge you to confront if you face it. Resist the temptation to deny its existence. Your first line of defense against depression is regular exercise—yet another good reason to stick to the program. If that doesn't put you on the rebound, you might well want to talk things over with your physician. Some of the newer antidepressant medications work extraordinarily well; unfortunately, though, some of the antidepressants themselves can interfere with erections, ejaculation, or both.

Medications and Erections

Many medications can inhibit the ability to achieve an erection, and if you suspect this problem, it's wise to talk it over with your physician. The common types of medications that are the big offenders include the antihypertensive beta-blockers such as Inderal (which is sometimes referred to as "end-it-all" by physicians because it can cause both impotence and depression); the antihypertensive Catapress; the diuretic hydrochlorothiazide, which is most often used in combination with triamterene in the antihypertensive Dyazide and its generic equivalents; various antihistamines; the antiulcer medication Tagamet; various antipsychotics; the antianxiety medications in the benzodiazepine class, such as Valium, Librium, and Xanax; digoxin (Lanoxin), which is used primarily in congestive heart failure and to slow down the heart in atrial fibrillation; the antiseizure medication Dilantin; and various antidepressants, which is a complex subject all by itself, because the lifting of the depression that these medications produce can dramatically *improve* sexual function.

The new types of antidepressants in the seratonin-reuptake-inhibitor class such as Prozac, Zoloft, and Paxil are not especially known for producing erectile dysfunction, but they can produce ejaculatory dysfunction, in which a man can achieve an erection but then has difficulty coming to a climax. They can also decrease the ability of women to achieve orgasm. To further complicate this subject, there is one antidepressant medication, Desyrel (trazodone), from the old tricyclic antidepressant class, which tends to *improve* men's sexual function independent of its antidepressant effects. It does so, however, at the risk of *priapism,* an erection that won't go down. (This condition sounds inviting but can actually be quite painful and harmful.) Desyrel also produces enough sleepiness in some men to make it a less-than-exciting potency medication.

Although the effect of various blood pressure medications on sexual function is hardly any secret, I believe that the reason too many men are prescribed hypertension medications that diminish sexual function is that too few physicians *ask* their patients about the effects of the medications they prescribe on their patients' sexual function, and too many patients suffer these effects in silence.

For men who do have high blood pressure, it is noteworthy that, in one small study of only eight men with erection difficulties, the antihypertensive Cardura (doxazosin), which is also used to treat benign prostatic hyperplasia, *improved* the sexual function of all eight men. This would make it one of the very few antihypertensives that actually seem to promote sexual function. Cardura is an alpha-1 blocker that controls blood pressure by opening up the arteries, so it makes intuitive sense that it would improve the functioning of the penile artery. With such a long list of hypertension medications known to produce sexual dysfunction in men, Cardura could gain greatly in favor if larger studies support this small one. Its happy combination of appearing to improve sexual function while decreasing benign prostatic hyperplasia (described in Chapter 10) could make it an excellent choice for men over forty. Other alpha-1 blockers, such as Hytrin (terazosin), may have the same beneficial effects, but there aren't yet any studies demonstrating this. On the other hand, a recent study showed that more patients taking Cardura developed congestive heart failure than those taking other antihypertensives, thus complicating the descision.

The other antihypertensive that has been anecdotally noted to improve men's sexual function is Calan (verapamil), which is in the calcium channel blocker class. Calcium channel blockers also act by dilating arteries and are often used in Raynaud's disease, in which arteries in the fingers become too constricted in cold weather and produce pain, so again these reports make intuitive sense.

If you follow the program set out in this book, your chances of achieving erections that will allow you to have an extremely fulfilling sex life—even if they are not necessarily as hard or do not last as long as when you were a teenager—are excellent. However, there will still inevitably be times when stress and fatigue will combine to defeat your best intentions. It's not the end of the world! If your lovemaking session is visited with this pesky problem, concentrate on what is going *right,* not on what is working less than perfectly. Be sure to truly "be there" for your lover. It's pretty frustrating, to say the least, for women when their lovers withdraw emotionally when they can't achieve an erection. Simply acknowledging what is happening will help to take the charge off it for both of you, and will open up communication. It's also important to avoid being a spectator by mentally observing your own performance. A relaxed attitude will serve you much better than a mental panel of judges evaluating your erection and holding up Olympic-style number cards with your "score."

There are plenty of ways to satisfy a woman in bed even without an erection. Many women actually prefer oral sex to intercourse, and many women can come to a climax more easily with stimulation from your hand than from your penis. Be creative!

Many men find that, if they have an occasional lovemaking session that doesn't result in a climax, the next time they make love—often even later that same day—they are that much more sexually excited, and a good erection and a very exciting climax then come easily. They have, in essence, "saved up." Although they didn't plan it that way, the initial lovemaking turned out to be the spark that got them primed for the fireworks later on.

A patient of mine named Jennifer told me that she and her husband, Tom, had evolved into a style of lovemaking that worked around the occasional times that he was too tired or stressed to achieve an erection or to have a climax. "Now that Tom's in his fifties, and especially with all his new responsibilities at work, sometimes we get started on making love but he can't quite finish. At first he used to get frustrated, but now we use it as a time to be intimate and communicative, and to just hold each other close. Then, the rest of the day, he's thinking about the nice time we had together and looking forward to our next chance to be close. And when that time comes, he's almost always turned on, and the erection and ejaculation come easily. It's almost as though the first time was the hors d'oeuvre. It's gotten to be a very natural thing for us."

If all of the above fails to get the job done for you, there are still five more "big-gun" solutions to the problem. The first, obviously, is Viagra, the most successful new drug ever introduced in the United States. As successful as Viagra has been, however, it is important to remember that at least a third of the men who have taken it have gotten little benefit from it. Many of these men might well benefit from some of the other approaches that are available.

One, on the market even before Viagra, is the drug Muse (alprostadil), which is inserted into the urethra or opening of the penis, about half an hour before intercourse is desired. This has proved to be an excellent option for many men, and in fact my patients sometimes ask me why anyone would use drugs injectable by needle (see below) when a much simpler approach is available. The reason is that Muse, like Viagra, tends to produce erections that are shorter lived and not quite as hard as those produced by injectable drugs. Individual experiences vary, but in men for whom these drugs are of benefit, an erection with Muse might typically last about fifteen minutes, while one produced with injectable drugs might last perhaps forty-five minutes.

If pills by mouth don't work, the next step is injection of a drug at the base of the penis, where it exerts a powerful dilation of the penile artery. The newest drug of this type is sold under the name Caverject, and is the injectable form of alprostadil, the same generic drug used in Muse. While men are often reluctant at first to inject their penis, the needle is very tiny, and the injection quickly becomes second nature.

This approach can produce surprisingly firm and long-lasting erections. I often tell my skeptical male patients the story of the British urologist and impotence researcher Dr. Giles Brindley, who made famous the earlier drug that was used for this purpose, papaverine. This story is difficult to appreciate, or perhaps even believe, without first understanding that urologists talk about sex all day long and are often extraordinarily open about sexual matters. In any event, Brindley was speaking to a group of several hundred physicians and journalists, both men and women, about the use of injected papaverine to produce erections. After his opening remarks, he announced that he was going to demonstrate that the drug worked even under the most trying circumstances. He then took off his pants, injected himself, and produced a rock-solid erection in full view of the spectators!

If Caverject doesn't do the trick, the old drug papaverine can be added to it, or even a third drug, another oldie but goodie called phentolamine. The three together produce a concoction, sometimes called "tri-mix," which will produce erections in 92 percent of all men with even the most severe erectile dysfunction—a success rate that has given it the reputation of being able to "bring back the dead." The downside in all of these injectable drugs, aside from the obvious one of the nervousness most men initially feel about injecting their penis with a needle, is that a minority of men experience significant pain with the injection, and a much smaller minority experience a buildup of fibrous tissue in the penis over long periods of use.

An older approach that may be on its way out now that drug treatments have become so successful is the vacuum pump, most commonly sold under the name Erecaid. This pump is, very simply, a plastic chamber that fits over the penis, with the vacuum produced by hand pumping, either by the man or his sex partner. It has been shown to produce excellent erections in more than 90 percent of men who had problems otherwise.

If all else fails, urologists can perform penile implants, either with a plastic rod that produces a permanent erection, or with an inflatable tube that results in a penis that can be pumped up on command.

Of all the men who have seen me about erection problems, only one turned out to be an outright treatment failure. He was an older gentleman with long-standing diabetes, sky-high cholesterol, high blood pressure, and congestive heart failure. Even he almost certainly could have benefited from the penile implant offered by the consulting urologist—an option he declined. This almost 100 percent success rate was achieved with very few referrals to urologists; almost all the cases were handled with the skills and training of a family practitioner. The days when advancing age meant limited sex or outright impotence for men are gone forever—for those willing to communicate and make an effort.

Women's Issues
(Required Reading for Men)

Women's sex issues are in some ways a mirror image of men's. With most couples I've counseled in their forties and fifties, it is the *woman* complaining of not getting enough sex—quite a role reversal from when we were teenagers! And that complaint is almost always coupled with a yearning for more communication, intimacy, and tenderness, especially in the form of cuddling.

Janine is a patient I see often in my clinic. Although she has a number of health problems, we almost invariably chat about those concerning her husband, Sandy. "I still love Sandy very much," she'll say, "but there's a lot of frustration going along with it. He's spending so much time with his work and his service club that it doesn't seem like he has time or energy for me. I really want more physical closeness with him, and I'd be thrilled to be making love with him every day, but he not only seems to have less interest in sex, but less interest in *talking* with me. I can't really get turned on without some emotional closeness, so the times when he 'wants it' are usually a turnoff for me. We're really in a vicious cycle."

Many women find that this role reversal leaves them feeling doubtful about their attractiveness. Having been accustomed in their teens and twenties to fighting off hordes of persistent men, women in their late thirties, forties, and fifties may find themselves concentrating excessively on the changes in their physical appearance.

Carolyn, a patient of mine in her early forties, told me that it had become hard for her not to obsess about her looks. "When I was in my teens and twenties, if some guy on the street whistled at me, it was just an annoyance. Now, the rare times that this happens, I actually appreciate it. It's getting harder to walk by a mirror and not count the wrinkles or get down on myself for putting on a few pounds."

Yet, in truth, men often find the experienced, mature, assertive woman very attractive. A patient named Dan, a thirty-nine year old who was at that time single and dating again, told me, "You know, like most men, I find those women in their early twenties sexually attractive, and I'm successful enough that I could find one to marry if I wanted to, but they often either don't seem to know what they're thinking or can't communicate it. There's just no depth there at that age. In a way, I find a woman with a few lines on her face and a more mature body more appealing, because I know she's going to be more intellectually stimulating and more open about what she's thinking and feeling."

The biggest concern for women in this age group is menopause. Although many women come out of menopause finding themselves feeling more confident, more self-knowing, more assertive, and just plain sexier, going through it is never easy. Despite all the new openness about menopausal issues, I've never met a women who felt prepared for the onset of menopause, and this is doubly true for women who go through the change of life at an earlier than average age.

Another patient of mine, Lisa, told me that, even though she knew her mother had gone through menopause at an early age, it still caught her totally unprepared. "My mother had told me that she'd gone through the change of life in her mid-thirties, but she never said much more than that. I guess she thought it was a private thing. The first time I missed a period, at the age of thirty-six, I thought I might be pregnant. Then I started to get really irritable, and then the hot flashes started, and I began to put two and two together. I'd already had my two children, so that wasn't an issue, but it just seemed unfair. It made me feel old, and I just wasn't *ready* to feel old. And it wasn't just the significance of the milestone, but the emotional swings I was going through with all the hormonal changes. For almost two years I was pretty rough on my husband. Sometimes, when I look back on it, I'm surprised he didn't leave me."

Many women go through a serious depression that coincides with the menopausal years. Along with the irritability and other symptoms of menopause, this is a time that can be very hard on a sexual relationship, even one that has been excellent for years. Communication is key and can be enhanced by a supportive health care provider or a relationships counselor. The mood swings and hot flashes can usually be treated successfully with estrogen therapy (more on this in Chapter 9).

Aside from menopause itself, women often find that their sexual concerns fall into two categories: self-doubts and body changes. It's possible to be in denial about the passing years up to a certain point, but when menopause hits there's a soul-searching that most women go through, along with long looks in the mirror to see if the attractiveness is still there. Yet this stage of life—what Gail Sheehy, in *New Passages,* has termed "second adulthood"—isn't about trying to look twenty years old, but about finding a new self-image as a mature woman, of realizing that the normal weight gain and the wrinkles here and there are a sign of acquired wisdom, not loss of beauty.

Steve, a fifty-one-year-old architect, told me that he found a new beauty in his wife, Megan, following her menopausal years. "When Megan first started having irregular periods three years ago, along with the crying spells, it hit her like a ton of bricks, even though, at the age of forty-seven, it wasn't entirely unexpected. We went through a tough eighteen months together, and with her bouts of depression and what-all, there were times when our sex life dropped off to making love only two or three times a month, a shadow of what it had been before. Megan somehow seemed to feel that she wasn't attractive any more, despite all my reassurances. And of course my own sexual responsiveness isn't what it was when I was twenty. When I was a little slow to get started, she saw that as evidence that she wasn't sexually desirable anymore.

"It took a long time for me to get through to her that I still loved her—more than ever, in fact—even if she didn't still have a teenager's body," he continued. "We've raised three wonderful children and gone down the road a long way together, and to me a few wrinkles and a few extra pounds here and there are badges of honor.

> **SIDEBAR 7.4**
>
> ## Testosterone and Female Sexual Desire
>
> Most people think of testosterone as a male hormone, but in fact women also produce it throughout their lives, although in much smaller amounts. In both men and women, it acts to stimulate sexual interest, and it may also affect sensitivity to sexual stimulation and orgasmic ability. In women, unlike estrogen therapy, which merely slows postmenopausal bone loss, testosterone therapy actually seems to *build* bone, so a combination of estrogen and testosterone may prevent osteoporosis more effectively than estrogen alone.
>
> Women who have experienced a sudden and unexplained loss of interest in sex, especially if it occurs after menopause, may benefit from testosterone replacement therapy in very small doses, which do not result in the facial hair or voice changes that higher doses of testosterone produce in men. It is usually administered via long-acting injection, skin patch, or cream, as it is very poorly absorbed orally.
>
> Women who are considering testosterone therapy need to get a spectrum of cholesterol testing to monitor the decrease in high-density lipoprotein (HDL, also called "good" cholesterol) that can occur with testosterone replacement.

"We talked and talked," he said, "and in time things got better. Now our sex life has really taken off again. The kids are out of the house, we have time for weekends together for the first time in years, and we don't have to worry about pregnancy anymore, or even those times of the month. We know each other so well, and are so much in tune with each other's bodies, that making love is like a symphony now. We've never been happier."

Many women, once the passage through menopause has been completed and the adjustments made, find that their libido and their passion have never been greater. On the other hand, women do experience sexual function problems that are in some ways like to the erection problems of men, as odd as that sounds. The clitoris is embryologically analogous to the penis, and a very early fetus has genitalia that are "ambivalent," meaning they can become either a penis *or* a vagina—in the latter case with a clitoris that is formed of the same tissue that could have been a penis. What determines the outcome is the Y-chromosome: Women have two X-chromosomes, while men have an X and a Y.

In many postmenopausal women, the same vascular effects of atherosclerosis that produce erectile dysfunction in men produce a syndrome whose symptoms may include decreased clitoral sensation, difficulty achieving clitoral orgasm, decreased vaginal lubrication, decreased vaginal sensation, painful vaginal penetration, or increased time for vaginal arousal. There is increased awareness in the medical profession that this syndrome is primarily one of vascular insufficiency, in which the vagina and the clitoris are not getting an adequate blood supply.

The first line of defense is the same old triad of diet, exercise, and a nonsmoking lifestyle. The second line of defense is estrogen replacement, not only to change the hormonal environment, but also to keep the vascular system in the best possible working order (which is exactly why postmenopausal women taking estrogen have far lower rates of heart attacks). Estrogen by mouth or with the skin patch works best, but for women who can't take estrogen by these routes or for whom vaginal dryness persists, estrogen creams applied directly to the vaginal wall can be extremely helpful. Even topical estrogen is absorbed to a certain extent; however, this may not be a panacea for women who have difficulty tolerating oral estrogen. Also helpful for intercourse are water-soluble lubricants, which these days even come in tasty flavors!

Most women find that, with the passing of time and their increased skill in lovemaking and lessening of inhibitions, orgasms come more easily and frequently. For those women who find otherwise, the most common reason is emotional—when relationship difficulties with a partner are inhibiting sexual desire or the ability to orgasm, partners will probably benefit from counseling by a trained professional.

For those women who seem to have an organic component to their difficulty in achieving orgasm, one of the most common reasons is recreational drug use or prescription drug abuse. Just as in men, women who drink too much will find their sexual desire and ability to achieve orgasm diminished, and the use of drugs in the benzodiazepine class, such as Valium, Librium, and Xanax, can seriously impair sexual function. Cocaine and narcotics such as heroin and oxycodone or hydrocodone (Percocet, Vicodin, Lortab) are also death on sexual function.

Some postmenopausal women who have difficulty with orgasms will benefit from *Kegel exercises.* These exercises were originally developed to prevent and treat incontinence, the inability to hold in urine, but they've since been shown to strengthen and tone the pelvic muscles used in sex, and thus promote sexual satisfaction and the ability to achieve orgasm. The exercises involve repetitive contractions of the *pubococcygeal muscle.* This muscle, the one used to hold in the urine, goes into reflexive spasms during orgasm and is responsible for a great deal of women's orgasmic pleasure. It is difficult to learn the Kegel exercises by reading about them, because it is necessary for your health care provider to verify that the proper muscle is being exercised. There are, however, biofeedback devices that can verify that the exercise is being done correctly. The Kegel exercises can be taught by most ob-gyns, by family physicians, and by most physician assistants and family nurse practitioners. Similar benefits to the pubococcygeal muscle can be achieved through ordinary exercise—fast walking, jogging, or swimming, among others.

Another new and high-tech approach to revving up a couple's sex life is the use of *pheromones.* It has been known for years that animals and insects attract one another through sexually stimulating chemicals; only recently, however, has it been appreciated that humans use the same reproductive strategy. Pheromones for both men and women are now available and have been scientifically shown to increase hugging, kissing, and sexual intercourse with the opposite sex. They can be obtained commercially through the Athena Institute in Haverford, Pennsylvania.

Sexual Fulfillment in Second Adulthood

With taboos diminished and more openness about sex than ever before, many people are now finding themselves single and sexually active at a time in their lives that wouldn't have fit the stereotype of a single person of that age even a few decades ago. And yet, despite all the expanding awareness of sexually transmitted diseases, studies have shown that sexually active singles in the over thirty-five age group are *less* careful about safe sex than today's adolescents! Part of this seems to be due to the current generation of adolescents' coming of age in an era in which AIDS has been a fact of their lives from the moment of their first sexual arousal, while their elders' carelessness may be due to the stereotype of people in their forties and older not being carriers of sexually transmitted diseases. It is vital to recognize, however, that those who are not in strictly monogamous relationships of long standing need to practice safe sex every bit as much as today's adolescents. Perhaps the MTV generation has something to teach us.

If we look around us, it's easy to find people in their forties, fifties, and even three or four decades beyond with happy and fulfilling sex lives. I'm tempted to say that they are as active as rabbits, but that's not the real story. What is far more important is that as adults in our prime we have the experience and maturity to maintain love lives based on trust, communication, and commitment. The depth of our passion and profoundness of our experience can go far beyond what we were capable of in our teens and twenties.

CHAPTER EIGHT

Children in Second Adulthood

Nothing in human experience is more primordial than the urge to procreate, the desire to give to our children what we ourselves were given by our parents—or often, even, to give to them what we did *not* have. When we love a child—probably the deepest and purest love we are capable of experiencing—the intensity comes from our knowing that this child is a part of us, that this child is our gift to the future, that what we bequeath to this child in love and support and caring is his or her beginning in the world. Children rekindle our wonder at the marvels around us and keep us young by bringing back our own cherished childhood memories.

One of the greatest privileges of being a physician is the chance to be present at the joyous moment that conception is confirmed and then to follow a couple through pregnancy and on to that most awesome and moving of human experiences, the miracle of birth.

And when the proud couple returns to the clinic, those magic moments of watching a baby examine her own hands, truly seeing them for the first time, or delighting in his beaming smile and spontaneous cooing as he recognizes his mother's face, make all the travails of being a doctor worthwhile.

Many of us now in second adulthood have raised our families, have a sense of completion and satisfaction about it, and are only too happy to be free and able to travel, do volunteer work, or pursue whatever adventures life has to offer. Other empty-nesters, having raised one family and perhaps having remarried, are now asking themselves, "If one family was that wonderful, why not a second?" Still others find that they have postponed childbearing far later than the previous generation and are now considering children at an age when many of their contemporaries are bidding adieu to young adult children. And still others find that they have become the primary caregivers to young grandchildren, usually because their own children have fallen victim to the ravages of drugs or alcohol.

There is no doubt that children can keep us young, that their link with creation and new life and wonder and joy is revitalizing and rejuvenating. And, with our new understanding of how to stay physically youthful much longer, many couples in second adulthood are throwing convention to the winds and starting, or restarting, their families.

A couple in my practice, Frank and Liz, seem to have started a 1990s version of the Brady Bunch. As Liz tells the story, "When Frank and I both got out of our previous marriages, I had two kids in college and he had three, and we each had a child at home: my fifteen year old, Todd, and Frank's twelve year old, Stephanie. With all those college bills, things were stretched pretty thin for both of us, and we ended up meeting at a laundromat, of all places. When we got married, at first we had no thought of having any more kids, but the idea grew on us, and when we had Jennifer, Frank was forty-three and I was thirty-nine. Having little Jennifer, who is now three, has been a handful, but she's really kept us young. When we go to the nursery school potlucks, most of the parents are twenty years younger than us." Every time they visit my clinic, they are glowing with pride at Jennifer's newest accomplishments, and I always look forward to seeing this broke but happy family.

Frank and Liz were lucky, but the ability to conceive, unfortunately, isn't always repeatable. The well-publicized media moms who have gotten pregnant in their early forties have caused a great deal of complacency among career women postponing childbearing. Men who postpone fatherhood are usually lucky; males produce sperm virtually throughout their lives, and men who become fathers in their nineties, though rare, are not unheard of. What *has* changed for men, other than the widespread postponement of fatherhood, is a dramatic decline in sperm counts, to about 50 percent of previous levels, in virtually all industrialized countries. There is strong circumstantial evidence that this decline is due to the widespread increase in meat consumption. Many meats contain concentrated pesticides—yet another argument for a diet that is primarily vegetarian.

By contrast with men, women who postpone motherhood are not so lucky, because women are born with all the eggs, or ova, they will ever have. Those eggs age, and they do not age well. There is a big drop-off in female fertility somewhere between thirty-five and thirty-eight, and for most women, conception is almost impossible beyond the age of forty-five.

Ob-gyns and general practitioners are finding that some women, especially high-achieving women who are accustomed to having a great deal of control over their lives, are in a state of denial about their prospects of childbearing late in life and hope that high-technology fertility treatments will give them the child they want. Most seem to realize the importance of amniocentesis after age thirty-five, as well as taking folate supplements while trying to get pregnant so as to avoid *spina bifida* in the baby (a condition in which the vertebral column is malformed), but few seem to realize how rapidly fertility drops off after the mid-thirties. In fact, of those women who are unable to conceive spontaneously and who seek help at fertility clinics, fewer than one in five will deliver. All will pay a staggering financial cost, which is usually not covered by insurance, and the majority who do not succeed will find themselves paying a heavy emotional price as well.

The aging of ova, however, is not the whole story. One of the unintended consequences of the sexual revolution has been a decrease in fertility rates because of infections in the Fallopian tubes, called pelvic inflammatory disease (PID). For fertilization to take place, the sperm must traverse the vagina, penetrate the cervix, swim through the uterus, and meet the ovum in a Fallopian tube. (To get clear on the anatomy involved, see Plate 6.) The fertilized ovum must then migrate back through the Fallopian tube to implant itself on the uterine wall. Anything that blocks a Fallopian tube will result in dysfunction for that tube and its ovary. Bilateral Fallopian tube blockages will result in outright infertility.

Pelvic inflammatory disease caused by gonorrhea generally, although not always, produces symptoms, but PID produced by chlamydia is most often symptom free, and either of these bacterial infections can cause a narrowing of the Fallopian tubes that can result in infertility. There are procedures to reopen the Fallopian tubes, but, for reasons not entirely clear to medical science, a surgically reopened tube does not function as well as one that has always remained open.

Ectopic pregnancies, meaning pregnancies that occur outside the normal site, the uterus, most often take place inside a Fallopian tube, which often requires surgical correction that will result in a dysfunction of that tube. In addition, a number of other conditions, such as *endometriosis*—the pathological migration of the lining of the uterine wall through the Fallopian tubes into other, inappropriate parts of the body—can also produce infertility, a risk that increases with the passing years. These various factors have combined to produce an infertility rate among American couples of traditional childbearing age that has now increased to about 10 percent, with much higher rates still among those beyond the traditional childbearing years.

SIDEBAR 8.1

Risks of Childbearing After Thirty-Five

Modern couples who postpone childbearing until later in life than is traditional are doing very well, on the whole, in part because they tend to be conscientious about seeing their obstetrician or family physician regularly and in part because they are less likely to abuse tobacco and alcohol. Nevertheless, there are risks in delayed childbearing aside from that of infertility, as discussed earlier. Almost all of them are associated with maternal age, not only for the obvious reason that it is the woman that does the actual childbearing, but also because older women bring much more genetic risk to the equation than do older men. While men create new sperm throughout their reproductive lives, women are born with all the eggs they will ever have, and as these eggs age, they become vulnerable to genetic defects.

Before discussing a few of these defects, let us quickly address the four most important other risks in delayed pregnancies: gestational diabetes, hypertension, the increased probability of cesarean section, and the increased probability of twin births.

Gestational diabetes, or diabetes that develops during pregnancy and then rapidly resolves after delivery, is a risk with any pregnancy, but more so with older mothers. In part, this is because diabetes is more common with advancing age under any circumstances, but it is also very much weight related even independent of pregnancy, and most women have put on at least a few extra pounds by their mid-thirties.

Hypertension in pregnancy falls into two categories: *essential hypertension,* meaning the everyday variety that is often worsened by the stress and weight gain of pregnancy, and *preeclampsia,* a condition that, if untreated, can rapidly degenerate to outright eclampsia, or seizures in pregnancy. Preeclampsia is almost always a disease of first pregnancies, but it occurs more often in women who are experiencing their first pregnancy after the age of thirty-five than in younger women.

Cesarean sections are more often necessary in older mothers, because labor generally takes longer for them as a result of the decreased muscle tone in the uterus.

Twin births, and even triplets and higher multiple births, are more common with advanced maternal age because of the increased likelihood of ovulating more than one egg with each cycle. Aside from the surprise of discovering an impending multiple birth when mom appears for her first sonogram, multiple births definitely fall under the category of complications of pregnancy because of the increased risk of premature deliveries, low birth weights, and problems with the placenta/placentas or umbilical cords.

Now let us return to genetics. All normal humans have a set of twenty-two pairs of *autosomal chromosomes,* whose genes direct the creation and development of the body in every way *other* than sexual characteristics. Every normal baby has one of each of these twenty-two chromosomes from the mother, and one of each from the father. Sometimes, however, an error occurs in which three of each set, rather than the normal two, are linked, a condition known as *trisomy.* The best known of these errors is trisomy 21, or *Down's syndrome,* in which the baby has three copies of chromosome number 21. These children will have low IQs in the 45 to 55 range, and one-third will have serious heart defects. On the other hand, Down's children are often extraordinarily affectionate. The risk of Down's rises sharply with maternal age, from less than 1 in 1,000 below age thirty to 1 in 378 at age thirty-five, 1 in 106 at age forty, and 1 in 30 at age forty-five.

With two exceptions, the other trisomies are so severe that they almost always result in miscarriages. The two exceptions are trisomy 13 and trisomy 18. Even these, however, are so medically serious that infants afflicted with these syndromes usually live only a few weeks or months. Both are more common with advanced maternal age.

In addition to the autosomal chromosomes, all normal individuals have a pair of *sex chromosomes,* which determine whether they are male or female. Those with two X's (XX) are female, and those with an X and a Y (XY) are male. Here, too, a number of errors can occur, but they are more survivable than those associated with the autosomal chromosomes.

The one sex-chromosome error that clearly occurs more often with advanced maternal age is *Klinefelter's syndrome,* in which a male has an extra X-chromosome (XXY), resulting in a normal-to-subnormal IQ, enlarged breasts (usually), and sterility. The average rate of occurrence of Klinefelter's is 1 in 500, but it is considerably more common in mothers over the age of thirty-five.

Klinefelter's must be distinguished from the unnamed XYY syndrome, which is well known even outside of medical circles because it results in tall males who are often unusually aggressive and therefore sometimes in conflict with the law. The XYY syndrome, however, does not seem to be related to advanced maternal age.

All women desiring pregnancy, regardless of age, should take a supplement of 400 micrograms per day of folate to help prevent fetal defects that can result in spina bifida.

All of this leaves couples who are beyond traditional childbearing age with much to discuss with their obstetrician or family physician and, ideally, with an expert in genetic counseling.

The bottom line is, first, that there are plenty of reasons in nonmonogamous relationships for using barrier contraception—such as the male or the new female condom, spermicidal foams, or the diaphragm or cervical cap—other than the obvious motivation of avoiding AIDS. Those outside the medical profession don't yet seem to have gotten the message that unprotected sex can result in long-term infertility. Second, many women in their mid-thirties seem not to realize that their fertility will not last forever and that if they want children, they would be wise not to wait—aside from the fact, of course, that the right relationship doesn't necessarily come along on cue.

The number of fertility clinics has exploded in direct proportion to the number of couples who have postponed childbearing long enough to find that conception has eluded them. The couples who go to these clinics will find a broad array of new fertilization techniques, all of which have in common high price tags and low success rates. And, while fertility drugs fail to work most of the time, in a few cases they work *too* well, as the world saw in December 1998 with the birth of the Houston octuplets.

These new high-technology approaches to fertilization late in life are largely outside the domain of the generalist. However, perhaps because of the very specialization of these clinics and their emphasis on cutting-edge science, they often neglect some low-tech but extremely worthwhile approaches to achieving pregnancy.

First, couples who want to conceive should have sex *often*. Fertility clinics tend to place tremendous emphasis on a woman's ovulation roughly ten days after the end of her period—a moment of fertility that is often heralded by a slight rise in body temperature—but this does not mean that couples should neglect having sex at other times. Having sex more often dramatically improves the woman's hormonal environment, and studies have shown that many infertile couples are simply not having sex often enough. An overemphasis on having sex at ovulation can make the sex clinical and joyless. More sex is better.

Second, women who wish to become pregnant should maintain ideal weight. Too high a weight changes the hormonal environment and can prevent pregnancy. Too low a weight can cause a woman to stop having periods and become infertile for different physiological reasons. The latter problem is one that plagues many busy, overachieving women who exercise excessively and obsess about thinness.

Third, to the long list of the pernicious effects of cigarettes, one can add infertility. Smoking has only a modest effect on fertility in women, but in men it definitely reduces sperm counts.

Fourth, infertility is yet another downside of alcohol consumption. Alcohol hasn't been shown to decrease the fertility of men significantly—other than by impairing their sexual performance—but a recent study has shown that women who drink even moderately have significantly lower fertility rates.

Finally, couples who want to achieve pregnancy need to relax. Stress is nature's way of telling our bodies that now is *not* a good time to get pregnant. Numerous studies have shown higher rates of fertility in women who meditate or use other stress-reduction techniques, and fertility rates are also higher in women who have a well-developed spiritual life, almost certainly for the same reason.

The result of the combined factors of couples postponing childbirth in favor of career advancement, declining fertility rates resulting from the sexual revolution, and a lack of knowledge or even psychological denial about how little medical science can do to help those women who have waited too long is an epidemic of "missing children"—of grieving for the children one has always dreamed of having but who never quite made the journey into this world.

The ultimate tragedy is the death of a child who *was* a part of our lives. We feel differently about losing an elderly grandparent who lived a full life and who will live on through children and grandchildren. When we divorce, as crushing as it can be at the time, we know that we can love again. The death of a child, though, is uniquely horrifying. In my emergency room, I have several times had to tell parents that their child has died in a car crash, and had to look into those faces of stark terror and see the gut-wrenching, fathomless void within. Most parents who have lost a child would bargain to take their child's place in death if they could. I'll never forget reading of the couple on an Amtrak train that plunged off a bridge who used their last ounce of strength to shove their baby through the window into the safety of rescuers' outstretched hands as the train car sank under the rushing waters and the parents drowned.

As tragic as the death of a child is, however, I have come to believe that almost as difficult to bear is the grieving for a child who never was. The world instinctively reaches out to console the parents whose child has died, but the barren woman grieves alone, mourning by herself the child who lived only in her mind's eye. Although she and her partner may be in mourning, their closest friends may be unaware even that they were trying to conceive. If the couple has given up trying, whether because of menopause or the exhaustion of their financial and emotional ability to continue with fertility treatments, the finality of their inability to conceive may be invisible to their intimates, who may make unintentionally hurtful comments such as, "There's always next month."

Many couples in the over thirty-five range are turning to adoption, but, with the competition to adopt newborn babies so fierce, these couples often find that their options are limited to older children from dysfunctional families. Most of us have a vision of bringing home, if not our own biological infant, at least a newborn we can know and nurture almost from the beginning of life. For some couples, however, fulfilling the need for a child means expanding their vision to include children older than newborns.

A few months ago, a woman in her forties came to my emergency room with her young boy, who had lost consciousness briefly when he fell on the playground and hit his head. From the outset, I was touched by the obvious love and closeness between them. She was Anglo and he looked Hispanic. She held his hand as he climbed onto the fearsome CT scanner, and when the X-ray series was developed, they marveled together at the 3-D view of his brain and how they could see his eyes and sinuses in cross section. She shared his childlike wonder at such miraculous medical wizardry. As I explained to her the symptoms of a serious concussion to watch for, she hung on my every word. And as they walked out together, hand in hand, I felt moved by her motherly love and their spiritual, if not biological, family ties.

My ER nurses recounted to me that the woman had endured a disappointing marriage to an alcoholic husband. Just at the time they divorced, she unexpectedly hit menopause at the age of thirty-eight, leaving her childless. In time, she adopted her little boy from a family with drug problems and found happiness in her devotion to him.

Several times in my work as a family practitioner, I have served as the physician to children institutionalized by Child Protective Services. As I've done physicals on children taken from their families because of abuse or neglect, I've asked them how things were going for them, and they've replied, "All right, but I want a mommy and a daddy," believing, in their innocence and simplicity, that the all-wise and all-knowing doctor could help them in their search.

It sometimes seems that those seeking adoption want a baby of a certain age, a certain sex, of their own race, and who is thought to be intelligent or gifted. But we are all God's children, and the less-than-perfect child who doesn't happen to look like us is every bit as lovable as the prodigy.

One of the primordial reasons for wanting children is our need to be needed, our fervent desire to make a difference in the life of a child. We sometimes forget, though, that adoptive children need us even more than the biological children we might have had. Blood may be thicker than water, but the strongest bond of all is the spiritual link between those who were meant to be together and who have reached out across time and space and somehow found one another. If you desperately want a child, I promise you, there is a child out there somewhere who even more desperately wants you.

CHAPTER NINE

Especially for Women

I often tell my female patients the story of Gilda Radner, the *Saturday Night Live* star who got too busy with her professional life to remember her Pap and pelvic exams and who, as a result, died tragically at the age of forty-two. To honor her memory, her husband, Gene Wilder, established Gilda's Club for cancer education and research. In an ideal world, all women would get a postcard once a year as a reminder to come in for a Pap and pelvic, but in the real world in which we live, it is up to *you* to remember.

The pelvic exam is no woman's favorite, but completing it faithfully every year will give you priceless peace of mind. The Pap and pelvic exams screen for three cancers: cervical cancer, ovarian cancer, and endometrial cancer. Endometrial cancer is not one of the most crucial to screen, because it usually heralds its existence with vaginal bleeding, but ovarian cancer and cervical cancer are silent tumors, meaning that by the time they produce symptoms, they have usually *metastasized,* or spread to other parts of the body, and can be inoperable. Catching these tumors in time can therefore be a life-or-death matter.

Women need to start getting routine health care at a much younger age than men because of the risks of ovarian and cervical cancer and of breast cancer. The yearly Pap and pelvic screening should be started at the age of eighteen or when sexual activity begins, whichever comes first. The reason that sexual activity is relevant is that the human papilloma virus in the male ejaculate is the primary promoter of cervical cancer. These days most women seem to understand the risk of AIDS from unprotected sex, but far fewer realize that cervical cancer is, in essence, a sexually transmitted disease that can be drastically reduced by insisting on condom use with occasional partners or by the use of a diaphragm, cervical cap, female condom, or spermicidal foam—and by early detection via regular Pap and pelvic exams.

Pelvic exams also screen for ovarian and endometrial cancer. The examiner begins by inserting a speculum into the vagina to open it enough to allow the cervix to be seen. After a visual inspection of the cervix, scrapings are taken of it with a wooden baton and a small brush that resembles a tiny bottle brush. The scrapings are placed on a glass slide and sent to a pathologist to inspect under a microscope for malignant cells—the Pap part of the Pap and pelvic.

The examiner then places one or two fingers in the vagina and another on the abdomen. The size of the uterus can thus be estimated, giving the examiner a sense of whether there may be endometrial cancer, a tumor of the lining of the uterus. The examiner then places the same two fingers under each ovary in turn by pushing the vagina to each side, with the free hand on the abdomen feeling the ovary for size and tenderness, a screen for ovarian cancer. Finally, in women aged about forty or over, the examiner performs a rectal examination with the index finger, as a screen for colon cancer.

Breast Cancer

Starting at the age of eighteen, women also need a yearly manual breast examination, which is usually done at the same time as the pelvic. The age at which annual mammograms should be started is controversial, although I believe there is now enough evidence to recommend starting them at age forty, rather than age fifty recommended by some authorities. It is clear, however, that women with risk factors—specifically, a family history of breast cancer or a known breast lump—need to start much younger, at an age that depends greatly on the individual risk factors, which should be evaluated by a health care practitioner.

Breast cancer is a scary subject not only because it is a common cancer, striking one woman in nine, but because it is so prone to metastasis. The incidence of this cancer is also on the rise, and although the reasons for that are controversial, I firmly believe it is because of the increasing fat in the American diet and because of our increasingly sedentary lifestyles. Breast cancer is clearly weight related, with the highest risk in women who gain weight in adulthood.

The *good* news, for those who need some reassurance before going in for a mammogram or a breast examination, is that the cure rates are also on the rise. In the 1960s, the five-year survival rate for breast cancer was 64 percent. The latest figures from the early 1990s demonstrate an increase in that rate to 83 percent. And it is also true that 90 percent of the lumps found during breast examinations turn out to be cysts or benign tumors.

Many women worry about the radiation exposure of mammograms. Especially with the new-generation mammography machines, the radiation exposure is very low, and study after study has shown that the benefits far outweigh the risks. Also, the new machines require less pressure on the breast and are not as uncomfortable as the old models.

For women in whom breast cancer is discovered, the available treatments include surgery (including both mastectomy and the less radical lumpectomy), radiation therapy, chemotherapy, and the hormone tamoxifen. The treatment options are very complex and must be tailored to each individual patient. For those facing these difficult questions, I recommend the book *Breast Cancer: The Complete Guide* by Yashar Hirshaut and Peter Pressman.

Menopause and Estrogen Replacement Therapy

Menopause seems to catch women unprepared no matter when it begins, but it can be especially jarring if it comes prematurely. Most women seem to think of menopause as being preordained to come around the age of fifty, but it's not unusual for it to start in the mid-thirties, especially in a woman whose mother and grandmothers had an early menopause.

At whatever age it comes, it is a shock. It is an incontrovertible milestone telling women that things will never again be as they once were and that the years of childbearing are now gone. It also brings the mood swings and hot flashes that can make it doubly difficult to bear.

The hormonal treatment of menopause has gone through a revolution in just the last ten or fifteen years. It wasn't that long ago that estrogen—most often sold under the trade name Premarin—was used almost exclusively in the first few years after menopause to quiet down the mood swings and hot flashes. However, while estrogen is unarguably helpful in achieving those goals, we now know that its far more important long-term effects are to decrease dramatically the risks of heart disease and osteoporosis while improving mood and decreasing depression. There is also strong new evidence that estrogen replacement decreases the incidence of Alzheimer's disease. For almost all women, estrogen should be taken lifelong after the onset of menopause.

> **SIDEBAR 9.1**
>
> ## Two New Drugs for Women Who Can't Take Estrogen
>
> There are now three new, nonestrogenic drugs that decrease the risk of osteoporosis, which occurs especially rapidly in postmenopausal women. Two act by limiting the absorption of bone tissue that occurs naturally as part of the body's ongoing renewal and renovation of the bones.
>
> Fosamax (alendronate) is taken daily in the form of a pill dissolved in a glass of water. Miacalcin (calcitonin) is inhaled from a nasal spray. Both drugs should be used with high doses of calcium replacement, preferably 1,000 to 1,500 milligrams per day.
>
> The good news is that both drugs have been shown to decrease dramatically the risk of osteoporosis. Fosamax sometimes causes some gastrointestinal upset, and, because of its poor absorption, involves the inconvenience of having to take it at least half an hour before eating. Otherwise, the known side effects of both Fosamax and Miacalcin are mild.
>
> The bad news is that neither drug decreases the risk of heart attacks or Alzheimer's, and neither has any effect on maintaining pelvic tone.

Before menopause, women have far fewer heart attacks than men, because their estrogen is protective and because, until recently, they smoked less than men. But after the menopause, and especially for women who smoke, the rate of heart attacks almost catches up with that of men. For women who take estrogen, however, the risk of a postmenopausal heart attack is cut almost in half. (In case you are wondering, when men are given estrogen, it is not protective against heart attacks, for reasons that remain largely a mystery.)

A recent study that received enormous publicity questioned the link between estrogen replacement and decreased heart attack rates in women. It is important to remember that this study is in conflict with numerous other excellent studies that came to the opposite conclusion. And the link between the onset of menopause—when estrogen levels plummet—and dramatically increased heart attack rates in women is established beyond question.

Osteoporosis is the loss of calcium from the bones; it strikes women past menopause far more seriously than men of the same age. It causes the "dowager's hump" that gives many older women a stooped-over appearance, and it weakens all other bones, including the hips and wrists, which frequently fracture in older women (see Plate 7). Estrogen dramatically decreases the loss of calcium from the bones of postmenopausal women, thereby reducing the risk of osteoporosis.

Estrogen also helps to keep the sexual organs firm and in good health, which, in turn, leads to a better-functioning urinary tract and fewer urinary tract infections. It also helps to keep the skin moist and youthful.

Finally, five studies indicate that estrogen decreases the risks of Type 2 diabetes and colorectal cancer, delays the worsening of symptoms of Parkinson's disease, improves sleep in women who suffer from insomnia, and improves balance and decreases the risk of falls in older postmenopausal women.

Unfortunately, though, estrogen replacement does not come without a price, mainly an increased incidence of endometrial cancer, a cancer of the lining of the uterus. Since this cancer is usually detected early through vaginal bleeding, however, it is not one of the big killers. The risk of endometrial cancer can also be dramatically decreased by adding progesterone (most commonly marketed under the trade name Provera) to the estrogen regimen.

Estrogen may also slightly increase the risk of breast cancer; the results of various studies on this are contradictory. Some recent studies seem to show a slight causal effect, whereas other, less publicized studies have shown either no effect or even a slightly protective effect.

To further complicate the issue, a major study has been released indicating that adding progesterone (provera) to an estrogen replacement program may increase the risk of breast cancer. The jury is still out on whether the link between hormone replacement and breast cancer actually exists, but even if it does exist, it is a weak link. It is important to remember that, whereas the average woman has a lifetime risk of 1 in 9 for breast cancer, her lifetime risk of heart disease is almost 2 in 3. The almost 50 percent reduction in the incidence of heart disease with estrogen use thus far outbalances any small increase in the risk of breast cancer—a risk that may not even exist.

My own sense is that many of the risk/benefit analyses that have been made of estrogen have focused almost exclusively on mortality rates. While virtually all these studies have shown that

SIDEBAR 9.2

Evista as an Alternative to Estrogen

As if the controversies surrounding estrogen replacement weren't complicated enough already, a drug called Evista (raloxifene) has recently been released. Evista is one of a class of drugs known as SERMs (selective estrogen receptor modulators), essentially "designer" estrogens. The other drug in this class that is currently available is tamoxifen, a hormone that has long been used as an anti-breast-cancer drug. Tamoxifen has been in the news recently because of new evidence that it may be able to *prevent* breast cancer as well as treat it.

Evista has been definitively demonstrated to increase bone mass in postmenopausal women, with no increase in the rate of uterine cancer. It has recently been demonstrated that, as a result of this increase in bone mass, fracture rates are decreased in postmenopausal women.

Evista has also been shown to decrease cholesterol levels. Whether this will translate into significantly lower heart attack rates will take longer to determine, perhaps several years. This is a vital issue, as estrogen has been shown to decrease heart attack rates by at least 40 percent.

A large study released in June 1999 indicated that over a three-year period, Evista decreased breast cancer rates in postmenopausal women by a striking 76 percent, placing this new drug in the class of potential blockbusters if more studies and more experience with it support this early promise.

As with estrogen, Evista increases the risk of blood clots. Curiously, not only does Evista not suppress menopausal hot flashes, as estrogen does, but it can actually *produce* them.

> **SIDEBAR 9.3**
>
> ## Advice for Women Who Decline to Take Estrogen
>
> Despite the consensus in the medical profession regarding the benefits of estrogen replacement, fewer than a third of all postmenopausal American women are taking the drug. Of the remaining women, some suffered intolerable side effects from estrogen, mainly fluid retention and breast tenderness. Some women find estrogen replacement unnatural and prefer not to take medication of any kind. Some women are too fearful of the risk of breast cancer to take estrogen, and if breast cancer runs in their family, the risks may indeed outweigh the benefits. And some women are simply not well informed on the issues or would prefer to avoid the inconvenience and cost of estrogen replacement for what might seem to be a far-off benefit.
>
> In truth, women who follow this book's advice regarding regular exercise, a nonsmoking lifestyle, and a diet moderate in protein will do better than average American women, because they will suffer less osteoporosis and heart disease. However, postmenopausal women who decline to take estrogen do need to make a special effort to maintain bone health.
>
> Aside from estrogen itself, there are now at least three drugs on the market that have at least some of estrogen's benefit. These are described in the two preceding sidebars in this chapter.

using estrogen comes out far ahead of forgoing it, that's really only one side of the story. The other side is the overall "youthening" effects of estrogen—the improvement in women's sex lives, the decrease in urinary system atrophy and urinary tract infections,

It is especially important for postmenopausal women not taking estrogen to limit their protein intake. When digested, protein is transformed into acid, with sulfur as a byproduct. The body uses calcium from the bones as a buffer to neutralize the acid, with resulting loss of bone density. For this reason, dairy products have an undeserved reputation for preventing osteoporosis, as the protein in milk will actually *accelerate* bone loss. The calcium in the milk may be helpful, but it is important to realize that, although osteoporosis is a disease of bone loss, it is only rarely a disease of lack of calcium in the diet. The relationship between dietary calcium and osteoporosis is a weak one.

I do recommend calcium supplements of 500 to 1,000 milligrams per day, but with the caveat that they are not central to osteoporosis prevention. Other supplements that may play a role in osteoporosis include vitamins C, D, and K and the minerals magnesium and manganese.

Aside from the extraordinary damage cigarettes do in promoting osteoporosis, alcohol is also known to accelerate bone loss. Refined sugar, salt, and coffee also seem to do this.

Finally, soybeans and alfalfa sprouts contain *phytoestrogens,* naturally occurring substances that have estrogenlike properties and that seem to quiet down the hot flashes of the menopausal years.

※

and the improvement in skin and muscle tone—not to mention the overall improvement in mood and sense of well-being that occurs with estrogen, long after the hot flashes and mood swings have ceased.

There are two basic philosophies about cycling estrogen and progesterone. The older practice was to replenish these hormones in as natural and physiologic a way as possible by giving estrogen on days 1 through 25 of the month and progesterone on days 15 through 25. This approach without question produces better bone health, as well as a more natural hormonal milieu, which provides numerous other benefits. Unfortunately, in most women, it also has the effect of restarting the menses at a time in their life when it no longer serves any purpose, but still produces the same discomfort and inconvenience as ever.

The more common practice now is to give both estrogen and progesterone every day, which usually does *not* have the effect of producing menses. There are still many holdouts for the older method, however, including many of the top researchers in the field, and the debate is not over. Although most women today who take estrogen supplements are on the more common regimen of taking estrogen and progesterone every day, exceptional patients who are willing to make the extra effort will want to discuss with their physician the more physiologic approach of cycling the hormones.

Women who have had a hysterectomy are often advised that they do not need to take progesterone, and while estrogen alone is the most common drug regimen for such women, it does not produce the optimal bone health and overall hormonal milieu that estrogen and progesterone together do. Ideally, even women who have had a hysterectomy should be taking cycled, rather than daily, estrogen and progesterone to most closely mimic the body's natural hormone production. Because of the complexity of this approach, however, it is the rare physician who is now prescribing progesterone for women who have had a hysterectomy, and it is even rarer to see cycled hormone replacement in a woman posthysterectomy. Nevertheless, there is strong evidence for cycling both hormones in women who have *and* who have not had hysterectomies. As more than one researcher in this field has commented, "It's hard to improve upon nature."

For women who experience side effects with the usual combination of Premarin and Provera, the most frequent of which seems to be breast tenderness, several studies have shown fewer side effects and more ability to remain on hormonal therapy with the more natural and physiological hormones, micronized estradiol and micronized progesterone. The first is sold under the trade name Estrace by Mead Johnson, and the second under the trade name Prometrium by Solvay Laboratories and by several other pharmaceutical companies in powder form.

Whichever regimen is chosen, all postmenopausal women should be taking calcium supplements. I recommend 500 to 1,000 milligrams per day. Unfortunately, even here there is controversy in the medical profession. Osteoporosis is a disease of calcium loss, so it would seem intuitive that replenishing calcium would prevent it. It turns out, however, that, within limits, the amount of calcium in the diet has little connection to the rate of progression of osteoporosis. It is important to understand that the three main risk factors in osteoporosis are a sedentary lifestyle, smoking, and lack of estrogen replacement postmenopausally. Calcium does play a role, but it is far less important than the other risk factors.

I have talked with many women who believe that taking estrogen or, for that matter, many other drugs is not "natural." Yet we're in an era in which hardly *anything* is "natural," simply because we're living much longer now. More than 99 percent of human evolution took place under circumstances very different from today's. Let's not forget that, as recently as a century ago, even in the United States, the average life span was less than fifty years, so few women lived much beyond the menopause anyway. Now that the average woman reaching menopause can expect to live at least another thirty years, there are excellent reasons for taking hormones that are found naturally in the body, in order that women may stay youthful and avoid the curses of heart disease, osteoporosis, and Alzheimer's.

There are a few "relative" contraindications to estrogen (reasons to consider forgoing the drug), according to the *Physician's Desk Reference.* One is a history of blood clots, a problem greatly worsened in women who smoke. The others are a family history of breast cancer or a patient history of liver disease, breast cancer, or gallbladder disease.

The most potentially serious of these is a history of blood clots, which can be fatal. On the other hand, the decreased risks of heart disease, osteoporosis, and Alzheimer's are so profound with

Especially for Women

estrogen replacement therapy that most experts feel the benefits far outweigh the risks, even in women who have had a blood clot—and the same could be said for a family history of breast cancer. The increased risks from liver or gallbladder disease with estrogen therapy are not great, and in my opinion should not be cause for much concern. Of course, you'll want to talk over the risks versus the benefits with your physician, but I would strongly encourage almost all postmenopausal women at least to consider estrogen therapy.

The issue definitely has an emotional component as well as a rational one, and I have had many patients who had such strong feelings about estrogen replacement that they declined it even after an extensive discussion of the risks and benefits. Adults have an absolute right to make their own health care decisions, and, as any competent and caring physician would, I respect the right of patients to make those decisions free of any pressure or judgment from others.

Aside from the pharmacological aspects of estrogen and of the three drugs discussed in the sidebars (Fosamax, Miacalcin, and Evista), there are two crucial lifestyle choices that may well be more important than drugs. Regular exercise, or even yoga postures that put the bones under a slight stress, will dramatically reduce the loss of calcium that results in osteoporosis. But the most important risk factor for osteoporosis is smoking, which *doubles* the rate of calcium loss from the bones—yet another reason for making smoking cessation the top health priority for any smoker.

Hysterectomy

An important question many women will face is whether to have a hysterectomy. This operation is done at much higher rates in the United States than in any other country, with more than a third of all American women undergoing the procedure at some point in their lives.

The decision is a complex one. There is more than one type of hysterectomy; often the ovaries or the cervix, or both, are left in place when the uterus is removed. The decision for a premenopausal woman, whose ovaries are still functioning, is a very different one than one for a postmenopausal woman. And there is certainly a psychological component. Some women want to preserve their uterus at all costs, whereas others, especially those who have had painful periods or premenstrual syndrome (PMS), are happy to see an end to their menses.

One of the basic arguments for a total hysterectomy (which includes removal of the Fallopian tubes and ovaries) is that it eliminates all risk of three types of cancers: ovarian, cervical, and endometrial. To those reasons, which apply to all women, are added the most common reasons for hysterectomy: *endometriosis,* in which the endometrial lining escapes into the pelvic cavity, causing pain with intercourse and painful menses; *fibroids,* which are benign tumors of the uterus; dysfunctional uterine bleeding; a prolapsed uterus, in which the uterus protrudes into the vagina; and severe PMS or painful or heavy periods.

If the ovaries are left in place during a hysterectomy, this will maintain the normal hormonal environment for a few years, but at the cost of a continued risk of ovarian cancer. In the absence of a uterus, however, the ovaries will eventually stop cycling in about 50 percent of women prior to the age when menopause would have occurred anyway. At menopause, the ovaries in *all* women, with or without hysterectomy, slow down considerably. Even "old" ovaries, however, are sex-hormone producers; at any age, their loss results in a significant physiological deficit.

Leaving the cervix intact with a hysterectomy is also an option. The main argument for doing so is that there is strong evidence that the cervix is a sexual organ. About half of all women who have hysterectomies report markedly decreased libido within two years, and the cervix is known to have nerve endings heavily localized within the tissue. A study done in 1983 in Scandinavia compared one hundred women who had received a subtotal hysterectomy, in which the cervix was retained, with one hundred women who had received a total hysterectomy, in which it was removed. There was a significant loss in the capacity to experience orgasm during intercourse in the group of women who had the total hysterectomy.

Despite the foregoing, conventional medical wisdom has long held that the cervix is just an asexual organ, one lacking in sensation. In my own medical school, we were taught that during endometrial biopsies, in which a probe is inserted through the cervix to sample the lining of the uterus as a screen for cancer, the

> **SIDEBAR 9.4**
>
> ## Women and Heart Attacks
>
> At all ages, but especially between forty and fifty, when most women are still premenopausal, men have higher rates of heart attacks than women. This is by far the most significant reason why women usually live longer than men. (The other big reason is the higher rate of lung cancer in men, although with more women smoking, that gender gap is narrowing. Perhaps the cigarette advertising slogan "You've come a long way, Baby" should read "You've come the wrong way, Baby.")
>
> Numerous studies have shown, however, that women who come to an emergency room with a complaint of chest pain as a result of a heart attack are far more likely to be misdiagnosed than men. This may be in part because emergency physicians are accustomed to thinking of this as a "male" illness, and in part because they them-

cervix could be gripped with a *tenaculum,* an instrument that looks like a long pair of tongs, except that it has two sharpened prongs at the far end. The theory was that the cervix was devoid of feeling. I do endometrial biopsies in my own practice about once a month, and am mystified how anyone can do this procedure even once without giving pain medication and conclude that the cervix lacks sensation. Needless to say, my patients get the medication. In any event, I have found that the tenaculum is often not necessary and that someone experienced in the procedure, with a little finesse, can usually slip the probe through the cervical opening, or *os,* without resorting to the use of such a barbaric instrument.

selves are overwhelmingly male and identify more closely with another male experiencing chest pain. Therefore, it is wise for a woman experiencing chest pain to be assertive and insist on a clear diagnosis.

Because it is more often men who experience heart attacks, and because it is most often men who are reluctant to seek medical care, the section on the crucial importance of emergency medical care for chest pain is in Chapter 10: "Especially for Men." However, it is no less true that women who experience chest pain need to be seen in an ER. Couples who are reading this book together might do well to have a heart-to-heart talk about the need for prompt action in any kind of cardiac emergency and about the potentially life-saving interventions available in your local emergency room if you are seen right away and a heart attack is diagnosed.

※

If so many in the medical profession haven't yet figured out that the cervix is a very sensitive organ, I have to wonder if the failure of physicians to recognize the sexual function of the cervix isn't another example of how a profession that until recently was heavily dominated by males has gotten on the wrong track entirely with regard to women's issues.

On the other hand, some women report *improved* sexual function following hysterectomy, with or without removal of the cervix, especially those who have had painful endometriosis or fibroids that have interfered with sex in the past. Some women also find that the complete freedom from worry about unwanted pregnancies is sexually liberating.

Although almost all women receiving hysterectomies in which the ovaries are removed are now advised to receive estrogen replacement therapy, there appears to be little question that this is not as satisfactory as the more natural hormonal balance achieved when the ovaries are left intact, ideally with the uterus also intact. Hysterectomized women—even those who receive estrogen—have higher rates of cardiovascular disease and osteoporosis than they would have had otherwise. They also have higher rates of urinary incontinence, in part due to the change in the hormonal milieu and in part due to the risks of the operation.

Finally, there is no question that women who have had hysterectomies have higher rates of depression than those who haven't, with the depression often not becoming evident until two or three years after the operation. Part of this is due to the change in hormonal balance, and part is psychological. Obviously, having the uterus removed is of tremendous symbolic importance and is a crucial milestone in the life of any woman. There is some evidence that the uterus produces its own supply of endorphins, which produce the "runner's high" in exercisers, and this may also be a factor in the higher rates of depression in women who have had hysterectomies.

Clearly, the subject of hysterectomies is complex. To any woman considering this operation, I strongly recommend the book *Hysterectomy: Before and After* by the reproductive biologist Winnifred Cutler, Ph.D. Although it is written for the lay reader, its subject is treated in such depth that it is a valuable reference for physicians as well. Cutler correctly points out that for women in the United States, the annual death rate from all reproductive cancers—breast, ovarian, cervical, and uterine combined—is only about one-eighth the death rate from cardiovascular disease (60,000 versus 485,000). And, when one considers the additional risks to hysterectomized women from osteoporosis and Alzheimer's, there are some very strong arguments for avoiding hysterectomy if at all possible. One argument that Cutler doesn't make, but that I would, is that the rates of hysterectomy vary tremendously from one part of the United States to another, leading me to conclude that there isn't much science in the recommendations about whether to have the operation. Cutler does conclude that hysterectomies are being performed in the United States at rates in excess of what is medically justified, and I agree.

Until recently, the medical profession was overwhelmingly male dominated. Although that has changed enormously just in the last decade, women still need to be especially assertive. We know, for example, that heart attacks in women are dramatically underdiagnosed compared to men. That, I believe, is due to the simple fact that cardiologists and emergency physicians are predominantly male and identify much more strongly with another man who is having chest pain. Of course, all patients need to be informed consumers and not be afraid to ask tough questions and get a second opinion if one seems justified. However, I believe that women may still be at a disadvantage in our health care system compared to men and need to be especially vigilant to make sure that they are getting the health care they deserve.

CHAPTER TEN

Especially for Men

Between adolescence and about the age of forty, men are in a different class from women in terms of the need for routine physical exams. Except for some of the "checklist" items in the next chapter—and with the exception of those who have symptoms of illness or who have risk factors such as smoking or obesity—most men up until the age of forty can do quite well without regular checkups.

Prostate Problems

Among the things that arise at age forty—aside from the need to screen for colon cancer, which also strikes women—is the need to screen for prostate cancer. This is the second most common cause of cancer deaths in men (after lung cancer and before colorectal cancer), and it will eventually strike one in ten American men.

> **SIDEBAR 10.1**
>
> ## Prostate Cancer Prevention
>
> Prostate cancer may be among the most preventable of all cancers. One of the primary—and controllable—risk factors for this disease is a high-fat diet, and there are therefore tremendous differences in the rates of prostate cancer throughout the world. The United States, for example, has *ten times* the incidence of prostate cancer as that of Honduras, where a much lower-fat diet is consumed. Even Japan, an industrialized country but one with a much lower-fat diet than that of the United States, has only one-fifth the rate of prostate cancer that we do.
>
> Prostate cancer may also be more preventable with antioxidants than most other cancers. Both vitamin E and selenium have been shown to decrease the risk of prostate cancer, as have foods high in beta-carotene, such as carrots and leafy green vegetables. Tomatoes, as well, have been shown to reduce the risk of this cancer (as well as many other cancers) through a substance called *lycopene*, which gives tomatoes their red color.

The prostate gland, located at the outflow of the bladder near the base of the penis, secretes seminal fluid during ejaculation. Plate 6 illustrates two important points about the diagnosis of prostate cancer. First, since the urethra passes through the prostate, men with this cancer will sometimes—although by no means always—have difficulties in urinating. Second, the location of the prostate next to the rectum makes it possible for the physician to feel it with a finger during a rectal examination. When cancerous, the prostate usually becomes harder and larger. The rectal exam is the most sensitive means for detecting prostate cancer, and, although it is one of men's least favorite medical procedures, it should be done yearly after the age of forty.

The blood test for prostate-specific antigen (PSA) is controversial. It definitely has its place, but as a screening tool it has limitations, because it can be falsely low even with prostate cancer and falsely high even without. Nevertheless, I believe that the weight of the evidence favors a yearly PSA test after the age of fifty.

Benign prostatic hyperplasia (BPH) is the noncancerous enlargement of the prostate that occurs with normal aging. In the United States, of men who live to age eighty, one in ten will require an operation, because of BPH, to open up the urethra and facilitate urination. BPH is not always easy to distinguish from prostate cancer, and the definitive test, a biopsy, has its own risks. As if that weren't confusing enough, there is a third illness, *bacterial prostatitis*—an infectious inflammation of the prostate—that has nothing to do with the other two, except that all three cause the prostate to enlarge. And, although all three can produce elevated readings in the PSA test, neither BPH nor prostatitis increases the risk of prostate cancer.

We now have at least three commonly used drugs to treat BPH. Hytrin (terazosin) and Cardura (doxazosin) are in the alpha-blocker class. Although both shrink the prostate, Hytrin is generally considered to be more powerful in this regard. Both will also decrease blood pressure, but Cardura is more commonly used for men with hypertension. If neither of these drugs shrinks the prostate, resulting in more comfortable urination, Proscar (finasteride) is often tried next. Proscar blocks the normal formation of a male hormone called DHT, a powerful stimulator of prostate growth. It does not decrease blood pressure.

If all three of these medications fail to produce comfortable urination, the next step may be either a *TURP* (transurethral resection of the prostate) or laser surgery. In both cases, an instrument is inserted into the urethra, and prostate tissue is removed, either mechanically or with a laser. Either of these procedures may result in higher rates of impotence, although it is controversial how many such cases are caused by the operation itself and how many have a psychological component. Neither the drugs used to treat BPH nor the TURP-style operations (including laser surgery) decrease the risk of prostate cancer.

If prostate cancer is detected, there are three main treatments: surgery, radiation therapy, and hormone therapy. Occasionally, however, the best strategy may simply be to do nothing. This is especially true for older men with a shorter life expectancy who have low-grade, less aggressive cancers and for men whose cancer is discovered too late, after it has spread throughout the body. In addition to getting screened for prostate cancer after the age of forty, men should be aware that the first place to which this cancer usually metastasizes, or migrates, is the lower spine. Thus, chronic back pain in older men should always be evaluated by a physician.

A classmate of mine from medical school, now a urologist,

recently remarked to me, "The more I learn about cancer of the prostate, the more questions I have about how to approach it." The complexities of evaluating the arguments for and against the various types of screening, and the various treatment options if prostate cancer is discovered, are beyond the scope of this book. For those who are interested, I recommend *Prostate and Cancer: A Family Guide to Diagnosis, Treatment, and Survival* by the urologist Sheldon Marks. The bottom line, though, is that men over forty need a yearly rectal exam, and it's important to let your physician know soon if you have any difficulties with urination.

The *good* news about prostate cancer is that, if caught early, it's 80 percent curable—an excellent reason to put up with those rectal exams and other minor indignities.

Another men-only cancer, testicular cancer, has been in the news recently, primarily because two sports stars have dealt with the diagnosis, one the beloved ice-skating star Scott Hamilton and the other the remarkable winner of the 1999 Tour de France bicycle race Lance Armstrong. Testicular cancer is so rare, however, that I have never seen a case of it, even during my training in referral hospitals. Nevertheless, a man who notices a change of any sort in his testicles would be wise to have it checked out by his physician.

Heart Attack

The other big difference between men and women after the age of forty is in risk of heart attacks. Men are at higher risk of heart

> **SIDEBAR 10.2**
>
> ## What Is Your Health Emotional Quotient?
>
> A huge component of people's health outcomes depends not so much on what they know, but on their Emotional Quotient—what they *feel* and what their *attitudes* are. Some of the following questions illustrate typical differences in the approach to health of men versus women. There are no right or wrong answers to these questions.
>
> 1. Regarding my attitude toward health issues in my relationship, I
>   a. believe that health issues should be a shared concern for a couple. The health of my significant other affects me and our relationship.
>   b. wish my significant other would stop bringing up my health issues. They're not his or her concern.
> 2. I see a doctor
>   a. for regular checkups and for any health problems that arise.
>   b. when the pain gets so bad I can't stand it any more.
> 3. My doctor diagnoses depression and prescribes an antidepressant. I
>   a. take the medication as prescribed.
>   b. accept the prescription, but don't fill it.

attacks than women at *all* ages—which is the lion's share of the reason why women live a few years longer than men, on average. But between the ages of forty and fifty, men are at *much* greater risk than women. The gap narrows once women hit the menopause, owing to loss of the protective effect of estrogen, but men are still at higher risk than women even after that point.

Especially for Men

4. My significant other shows me a mole that has gotten larger recently. I
   a. advise him or her to get it checked out right away.
   b. tell him or her it's probably nothing, and to mention it at next year's checkup.
5. My boss harshly criticizes my work. I
   a. feel down and question my self-worth.
   b. feel angry and spend the afternoon target shooting at the rifle range.
6. My doctor tells me that both my blood pressure and my cholesterol have jumped since the last checkup, and she is worried. I
   a. look to my significant other for support.
   b. say nothing, because I don't want to bother anyone.
7. With regard to the medications I'm taking, I
   a. know the names and the dosages and why I'm taking them.
   b. know that one of the pills is green, one is red, and then there's a little blue one.
8. I am a diabetic. My doctor tells me that if I don't change from pills to insulin, I will take five years off my expected life span. I
   a. reluctantly learn to self-inject insulin.
   b. decide I would rather die five years sooner than use needles.

※

Unfortunately, it's also often men who are more in denial about heart attacks. These days, we can usually break up the clots that cause heart attacks with potent blood thinners such as tissue plasminogen activator (TPA) or streptokinase, or with emergency angioplasty ("balloons"), but it needs to be done *as soon as possible*. Heart attacks come with a huge range of symptoms, all the way from crushing chest pain to mild discomfort to "indigestion" that is centered in the upper abdomen, and roughly one heart attack in six is silent—meaning the victim has no symptoms at all. The classic symptoms are chest pain, especially if it radiates to the arms or into the neck or chin, nausea or vomiting, sweatiness, and shortness of breath. Unfortunately, there are also plenty of nonclassic symptoms, including that "indigestion." Both men and women who have any symptoms of a heart attack need to go to an emergency room without delay.

Especially for those of us who are health-conscious and believe we've done everything possible to reduce the risk of a heart attack, it's all too easy to be in denial about "the big one." And even if we eat right and exercise every day, heart attacks are still a risk. Studies have shown that people with known heart disease—previous heart attacks or angina—are actually *less* likely to come in promptly to the ER than the population at large. If you're having any symptoms that even conceivably could be a heart attack, you need to see a physician. Be assured that your emergency room doc will take you seriously if you think you might be having a heart attack and that you'll get the electrocardiogram you need.

CHAPTER ELEVEN

A Checklist of Preventive Medicine

A number of important health topics don't fall neatly under any one heading, so this chapter is a catchall for those not covered elsewhere in the book. Most of these disorders are potentially life-threatening, so I hope you will not neglect any of their symptoms and wish you hadn't. There is much to be said for the peace of mind—not to mention the good health—that results from conscientiously addressing these matters.

Blood Pressure

Both men and women should get their blood pressure checked every year, unless they have hypertension and need to get it checked more often. This doesn't necessarily have to be done in a doctor's office, but if you take your blood pressure at home with your own cuff, be sure to bring it in and have it checked against a blood pressure device of known accuracy.

Don't forget that high blood pressure—often called the "silent killer"—usually produces no symptoms *at all* and can cause enormous damage that is usually irreversible. A partial list of some of the consequences of uncontrolled hypertension includes heart attacks, strokes, congestive heart failure, kidney failure, eye damage, and sexual dysfunction.

Cholesterol

Both men and women should have their cholesterol screened at least once in early adulthood. This is especially important for those for whom high cholesterol levels run in the family. Those who are found to have high levels will need to have their cholesterol monitored appropriately and treated, if necessary, by a health professional. Those with normal cholesterol levels will still benefit from repeat checks every two years after age forty.

Colon Cancer

Colon cancer is a seldom discussed disease that was in the news recently because of the death of beloved cartoonist Charles Schulz. In 1992, the world mourned the death of actress Audrey Hepburn from colon cancer. And in 1998, the well-known co-host of the *Today* show, Jay Monahan, died of colon cancer at the tragically young age of forty-two. To honor his memory, his wife, Katie Couric has launched a campaign to publicize this deadly disease that is highly preventable. Colon cancer is the third largest cause of cancer mortality in both men and women, after lung and prostate cancer in men and lung and breast cancer in women. Colon cancer is notorious for metastasizing to the liver, at which point it is almost always inoperable and terminal. Yet, despite its large number of victims, it hasn't received anywhere near the attention some of the other cancers have.

It is caused by carcinogens in the stool, and its incidence may be reduced through a high-fiber diet, meaning lots of fruits and vegetables, and bran cereal or oatmeal for breakfast. The extra bulk in the stool decreases the concentration of the carcinogens, and a bulkier stool also transits the intestines much faster than a low-fiber, less bulky stool, again decreasing the exposure. A low-fat diet also decreases the risk of colon cancer. Primitive tribes that eat low-fat, high-fiber diets have far lower rates of colon cancer than those of us who live in "advanced" societies.

When it comes to screening for colon cancer, almost all authorities agree that both men and women over forty years old should receive a yearly digital rectal examination, through which the examiner can feel tumors in the last few inches of the colon and the rectum. For women, this is usually done in conjunction with the Pap and pelvic exams; for men, the rectal examination serves *two* purposes in screening for both colon cancer and prostate cancer.

In addition, the American Cancer Society recommends that men and women undergo *colonoscopy,* a viewing of the colon through a fiber-optic device, starting at age fifty and every ten years thereafter. In practice, however, only a minority of physicians follow that recommendation. The patients don't like such an uncomfortable examination, doctors rarely have time to do it on all their patients, and it carries a small but real risk of perforation of the colon.

It also has a questionable cost/benefit ratio. Doing colonoscopies on every patient in the United States every year would increase the average life expectancy by a few months in comparison with the benefits of a yearly digital rectal examination and stool testing—but at a very high cost in time and money. On the other hand the lost years of life are not a few months per person, but rather *no* lost years of life for most, versus ten to twenty years lost for those whose colon cancer is diagnosed too late as a result of not getting routine colonoscopies. It is therefore hard to argue with those who recommend strictly following the American Cancer Society guidelines.

The other commonly used screening tool is testing three stool samples for fecal occult (hidden) blood, which is commonly found in the stool of those with colon tumors or their precursors, polyps of the colon. That test, however, is also controversial because of the high number of false positives and false negatives. Once these false positives are uncovered, the physician is under pressure to order a lot of expensive tests, some of which carry small but real risks. On the whole, though, the evidence for yearly fecal occult blood testing is strong, and I recommend it for those over age forty.

Low Thyroid

The thyroid is a gland in the forward part of the neck that secretes hormones that keep you energized and promote heat regulation. After the age of fifty, low thyroid, or *hypothyroidism,* is relatively common—more so in women than in men. There is increasing evidence that thyroid function should be checked every few years after age forty via a simple blood test for thyroid-stimulating hormone, or TSH. This is especially important if you note any of the symptoms of hypothyroidism: low energy, cold intolerance, hair loss, dry skin, weight gain, or constipation. Aside from the downside of these symptoms, low thyroid is a risk factor for heart attacks. Correction of low thyroid can result in amazing stores of new energy, and it often reverses the weight gain of patients who didn't realize they had this condition.

Diabetes

One of the latest recommendations of the U.S. Public Health Service's Centers for Disease Control is a "fasting glucose" test every three years after the age of forty-five, as a screen for diabetes. Those who have symptoms of diabetes—frequent urination, unusual thirstiness, dizziness, or blurry vision—should get a fasting glucose whenever the symptoms come up, especially if this disease runs in the family.

It is crucial to know if you have diabetes because, if uncontrolled, it can do severe damage to your cardiovascular and nervous systems. We are seeing an epidemic of new adult-onset diabetes[*] caused by the increase in obesity in our society, so for the person who does *not* have diabetes, the defense is twofold: diet and exercise, as always, and screen for diabetes after the age of forty-five. For those of you who would like to know more about diabetes, especially if you have it, I recommend the *American Diabetes Association Complete Guide to Diabetes* by Richard Kahn, Ph.D.

Skin Cancer

Finally, let's talk about sun exposure. It wasn't that long ago that getting lots of sun was believed to be healthy, and, in truth, too *little* sun can cause low levels of vitamin D. We now know beyond any reasonable doubt, however, that sun exposure is one of the principal culprits in premature aging and, more importantly, skin cancer.

There are three major types of skin cancers: basal-cell carcinomas, squamous-cell carcinomas, and melanomas (see Plate 8). Of the three, melanomas are by far the most feared, because they are, along with breast cancer, among the most aggressive of cancers and are notorious for metastasizing quickly throughout the body. All three skin cancers have more than doubled in incidence during the

---

[*]We are in the midst of a change in terminology about diabetes. Type I has been known in the past as insulin-dependent or juvenile-onset diabetes. Type II has been known as non-insulin-dependent or adult-onset diabetes. The new terminology is simply Type 1 and Type 2, in part because insulin is often used in Type 2 diabetes and in part because it is easy to misread Type II as "type eleven."

last few decades, as we Americans spend a greater percentage of our leisure time in the sun. Any suspicious wart, mole, or lesion on the skin should be inspected by your doctor, but the most worrisome ones are the fast-growing lesions, the multicolored ones, especially with blue or purple tints, and those with irregular borders.

It's hard to overemphasize how much the sun ages our skin. I spend a fair amount of my time in long-term care facilities with senior citizens, and as I do their monthly exams I never fail to be impressed that, no matter how wrinkled their faces and necks may be, their buttocks are almost always as smooth as a baby's—because they've never been sun-exposed—and even their torsos, below the collar line, have much younger-looking skin. Until recently, the prevailing wisdom was that facial wrinkles occur more often than wrinkles on other parts of the body, but we now know that the primary cause of almost *all* wrinkles is sun exposure.

I did my dermatology training in New Zealand, the melanoma capital of the world because of the high proportion of fair-skinned people of Irish and Scottish descent who cook themselves on the beach day after day, and I got to be quite expert at spotting and removing melanomas. I also came away impressed by the damage the sun can do. I myself don't go out the door anymore during the day without at least sunscreen.

There are many other minor modifications to your lifestyle that will make a huge difference in your sun exposure. If you're eating lunch on an outdoor terrace, for example, park yourself in the shade rather than the sun, and save yourself a few wrinkles. If you spend more than a trivial amount of time in your car, I recommend semitransparent shades for the side windows. (In the past it was believed that the more dangerous kind of sunlight was absorbed by glass, but there is new evidence that glass may not provide such good protection after all.) If you're touring the Acropolis in Athens on a hot summer day, stand in the shade under one of the pillars rather than in the sun while you're listening to the tour guide, and block out a few rays.

The *good* news about the sun is that there's new evidence that the damage it causes is partly reversible through decreasing our exposure. To me, that's a metaphor for all that we're learning about reversing disease processes. It seems that hardly a month goes by when there isn't a report in one of the medical journals about how an illness that was thought to be chronic and unrelenting turns out to be amenable to lifestyle changes. Even if you've exposed yourself to too much sun for too long in your backyard in Phoenix or Miami, once you start getting serious about avoiding the sun's rays, we now know that you can turn back the clock at least a little.

And that's true of almost *any* aspect of your health. Almost all of us have done things in the past that we now regret, whether it be sun exposure, smoking, drinking, drugs, a poor diet, or whatever, so we're all in the same boat in that way. The past is no longer in your control, so concentrate on what you *can* control—the here and now—and optimize your lifestyle to make the years to come the best years of your life.

CHAPTER TWELVE

The Evidence for Health Supplements

In recent years a number of health supplements have received press coverage, much of it uncritical or even biased. Some of these supplements are intended to promote youthfulness, some to restore energy and vitality, and some to act as preventive measures against heart attacks and cancers. Some are clearly beneficial, some are unproved, and a few may do more harm than good.

The "gold standard" in the medical profession for any therapy is the prospective, controlled, randomized, double-blind, statistically significant, repeatable study. What it takes to pass this test is a therapy that *really* works, as opposed to one that some doctors simply *believe* works.

The history of medicine is filled with treatments that were used for years because "everyone knew" they worked. For years, heart attack patients were forced into strict bed rest, sometimes even with nurses spoon-feeding them, until it was discovered that this treatment dramatically increased the risk of blood clots in the legs and of pneumonia—not to mention the psychological risk of the patients' assuming the sick role and becoming cardiac cripples. For years, when doctors delivered a baby, they would hold it upside down and slap it on the back to "make" it start breathing and cry—until it was discovered that newborn babies started breathing and cried without any assistance from the medical profession. For years, tonsilectomies were performed on children because it had been "proved" that they decreased sore throats and ear infections. Only after careful studies were done was it discovered that as children grew older, sore throats and ear infections plummeted whether they'd had a tonsilectomy or not.

A *prospective* study means that only patients who have not previously been treated are enrolled in the study; if patients who have already been treated were to be included, the results might be skewed. For example, more highly educated patients might be more likely to seek a given treatment, and, since they tend to have better health than more poorly educated patients, this could be the reason for better outcomes, rather than the treatment itself.

A *controlled* study is one in which the patients are divided into two groups of roughly equal size: One group gets the actual treatment and the other gets a placebo—a sugar pill—because we know that some patients will feel better simply from having gotten a pill of *any* kind from a health care professional. (This is called the placebo effect, which I discussed briefly in Chapter 5.)

Vulnerable Points in the Cardiovascular System

Plate 1

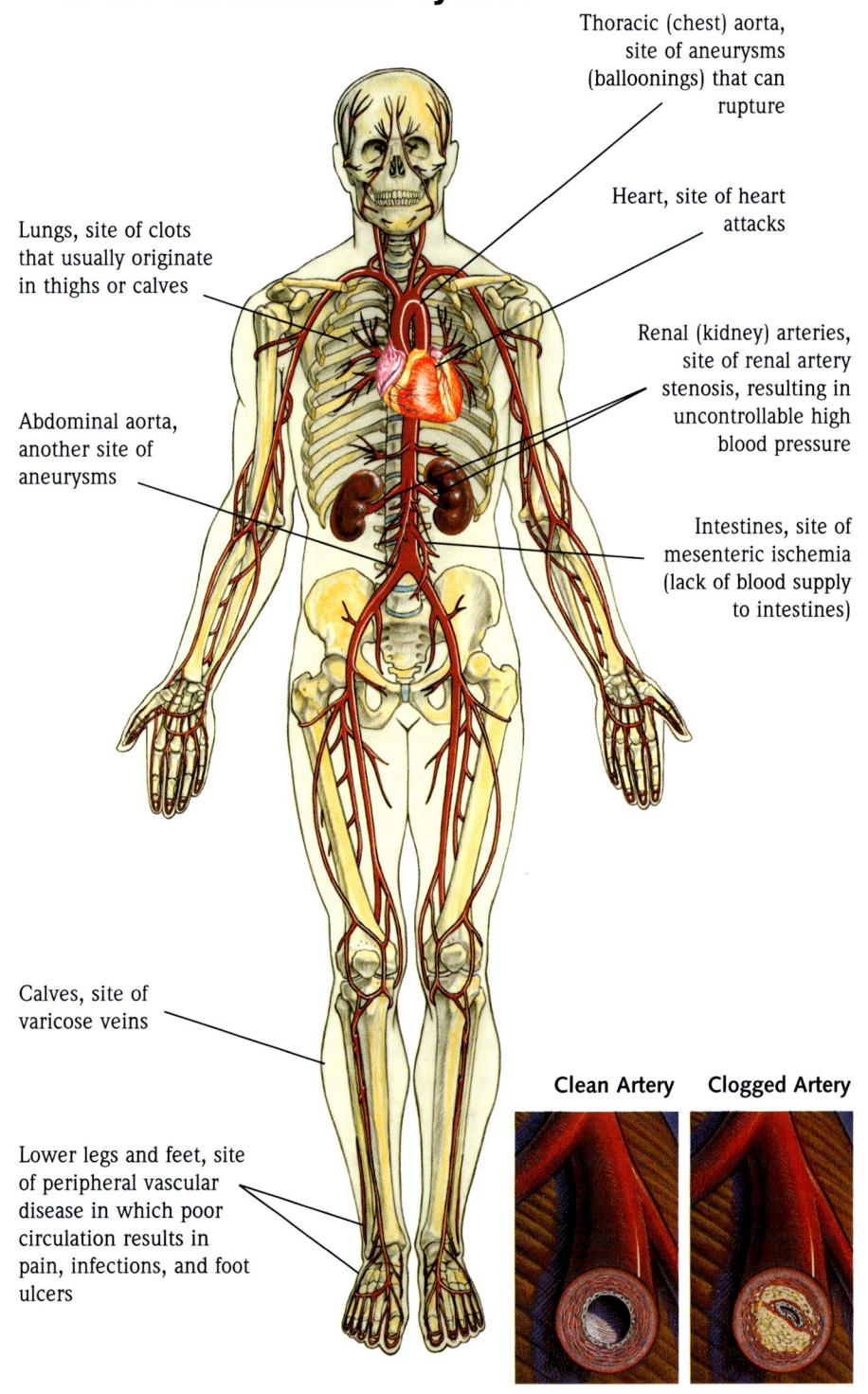

Thoracic (chest) aorta, site of aneurysms (balloonings) that can rupture

Heart, site of heart attacks

Lungs, site of clots that usually originate in thighs or calves

Renal (kidney) arteries, site of renal artery stenosis, resulting in uncontrollable high blood pressure

Abdominal aorta, another site of aneurysms

Intestines, site of mesenteric ischemia (lack of blood supply to intestines)

Calves, site of varicose veins

Clean Artery **Clogged Artery**

Lower legs and feet, site of peripheral vascular disease in which poor circulation results in pain, infections, and foot ulcers

Pumping Action of the Heart

Plate 2

Electrical Conduction System of the Heart

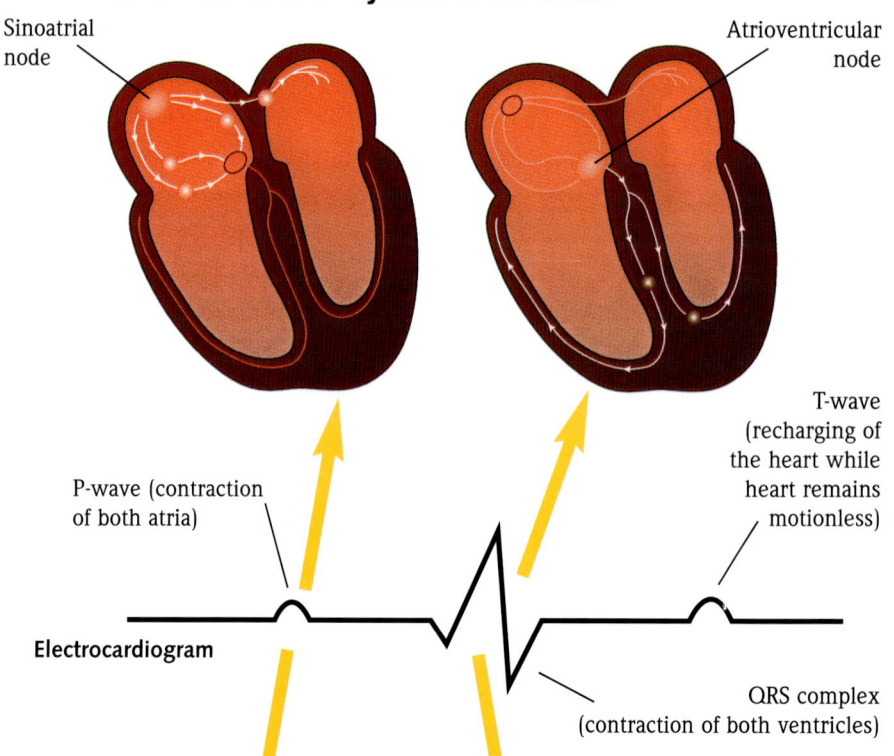

Sinoatrial node

Atrioventricular node

P-wave (contraction of both atria)

T-wave (recharging of the heart while heart remains motionless)

Electrocardiogram

QRS complex (contraction of both ventricles)

Blood Flow Through the Heart

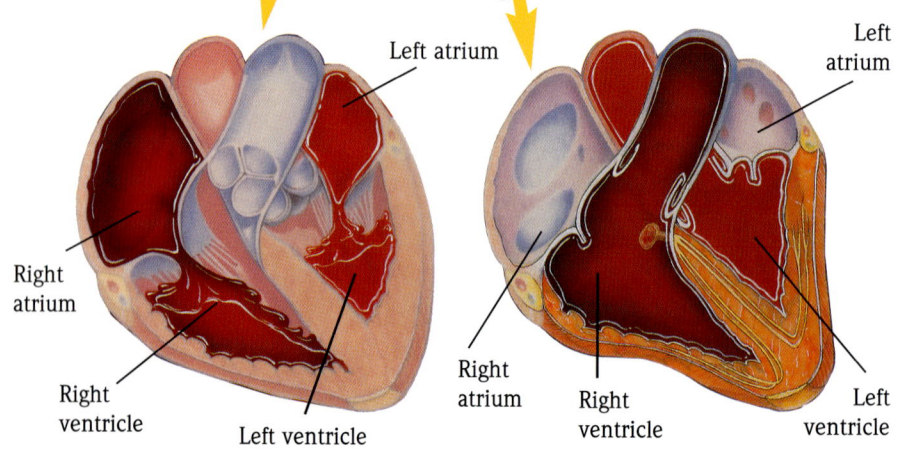

Left atrium

Left atrium

Right atrium

Right atrium

Right ventricle

Right ventricle

Left ventricle

Left ventricle

Following the electrical signal from the sinoatrial node, both atria contract together "priming the pump" for the two ventricles.

The atrioventricular node relays the signal to the ventricles which also contract together.

Blood Supply to Heart's Electrical Conduction System

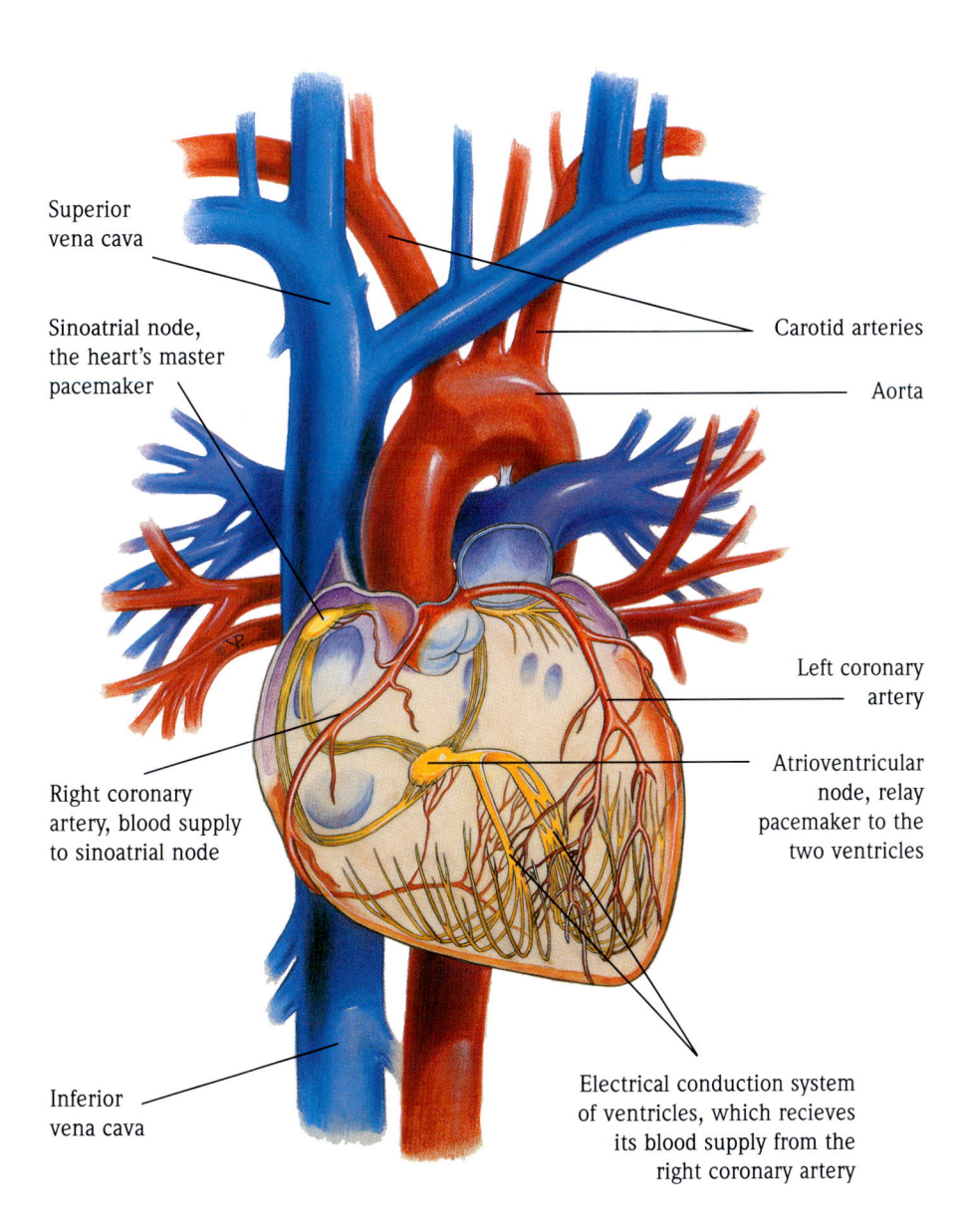

Plate 3

- Superior vena cava
- Sinoatrial node, the heart's master pacemaker
- Carotid arteries
- Aorta
- Left coronary artery
- Atrioventricular node, relay pacemaker to the two ventricles
- Right coronary artery, blood supply to sinoatrial node
- Inferior vena cava
- Electrical conduction system of ventricles, which recieves its blood supply from the right coronary artery

Heart attacks are caused by complete blockages in the coronary arteries, which will result in a permanent loss of heart muscle. Lesser blockages in the coronary arteries can cause angina or bad heart rhythms such as atrial fibrillation, atrial flutter, or sick sinus syndrome.

Blood Supply of the Brain

Plate 4

Ophthalmic artery (to eyes)

Circle of Willis

Carotid artery

Vertebral artery

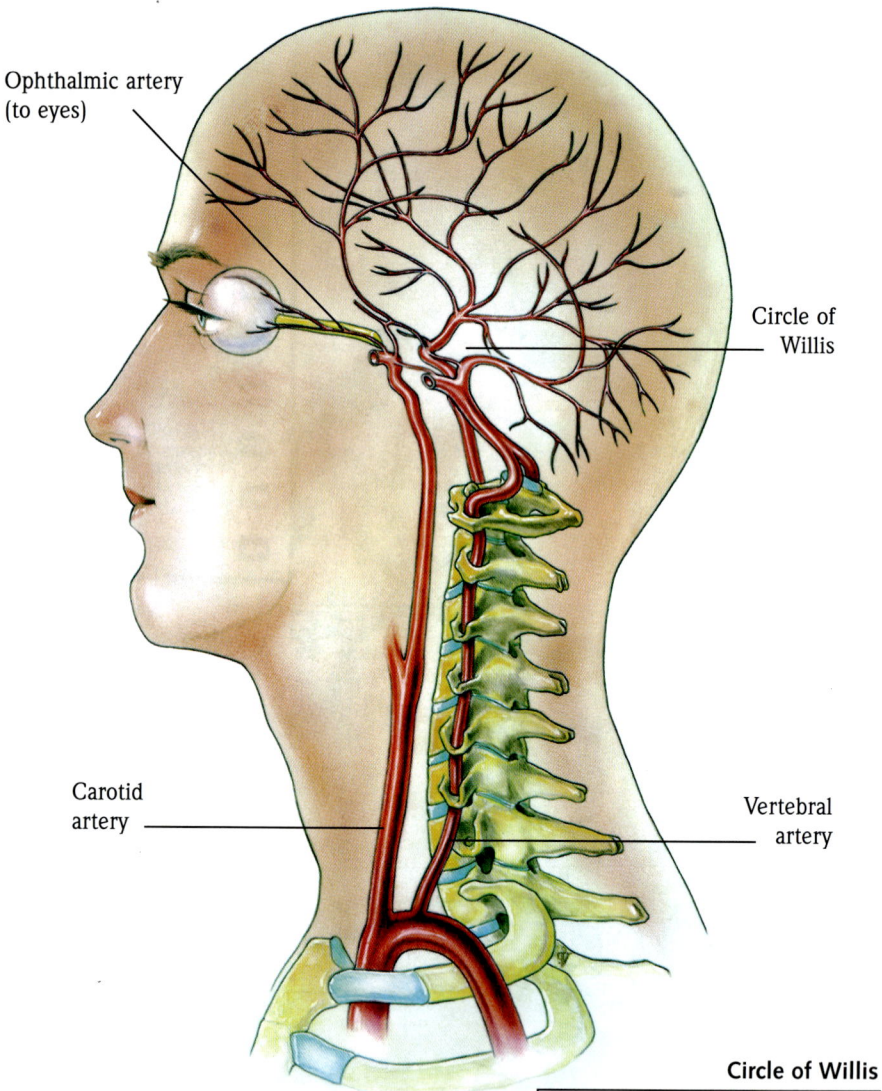

The brain is supplied by four arteries: two carotid arteries and two vertebral arteries which are threaded through small holes in the vertebral bodies that make up the cervical spine. The four arteries meet in the Circle of Willis and supply the blood inflow to this true circle. The remaining arteries in the Circle of Willis are outflowing arteries to the brain.

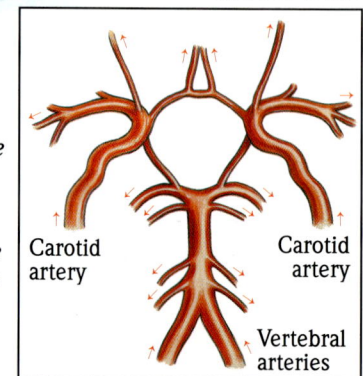

Circle of Willis

Carotid artery

Carotid artery

Vertebral arteries

Female Reproductive System

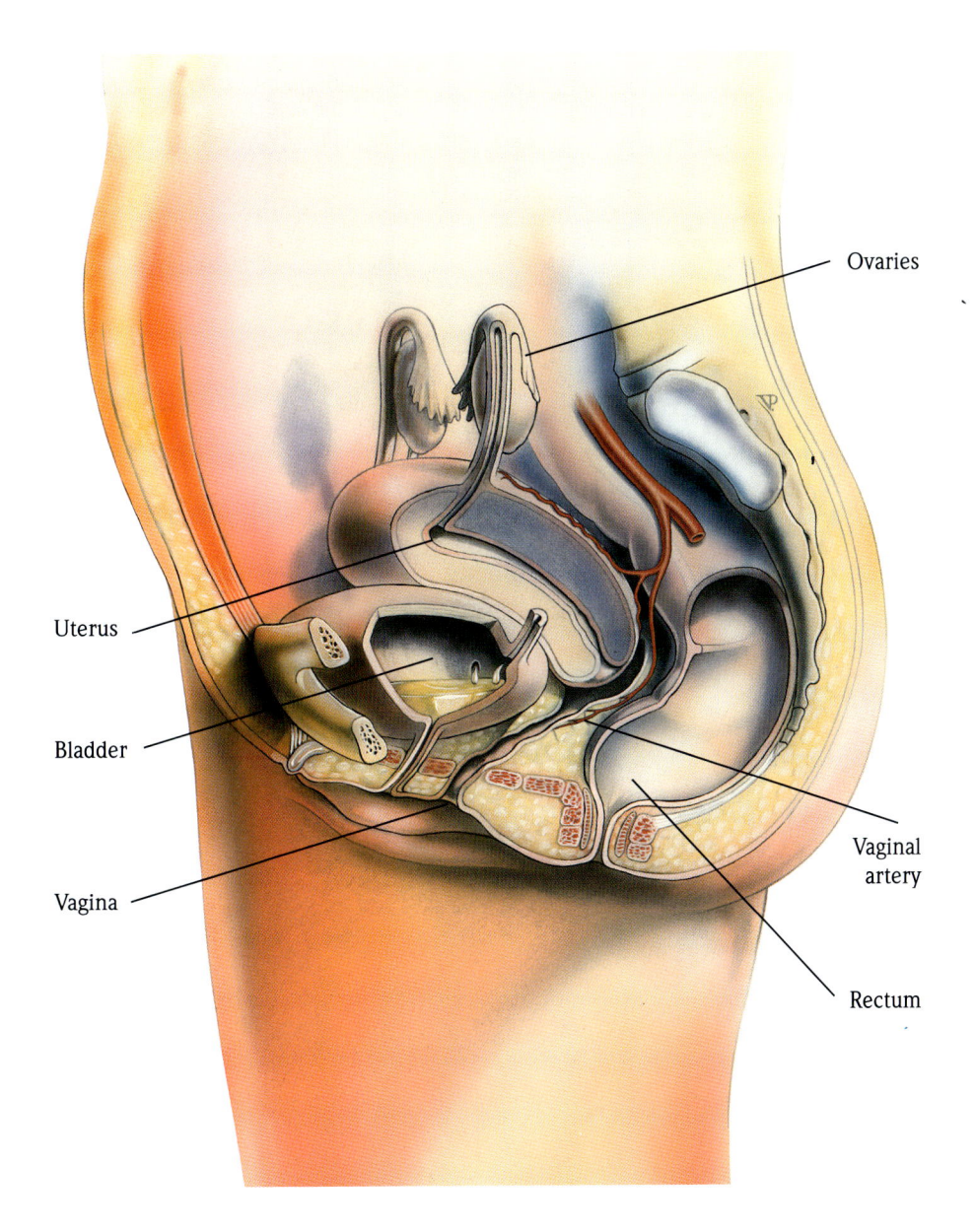

Plate 5

- Ovaries
- Uterus
- Bladder
- Vagina
- Vaginal artery
- Rectum

During a pelvic examination the physician will look at the cervix, take a Pap smear, and feel the ovaries and uterus for lumps or other irregularities. Good cardiovascular health will help to insure continued pleasurable sensation in the clitoris and vagina, as well as continued good lubrication during intercourse.

Male Reproductive System

Plate 6

Bladder

Penis

Penile artery

Rectum

Prostate

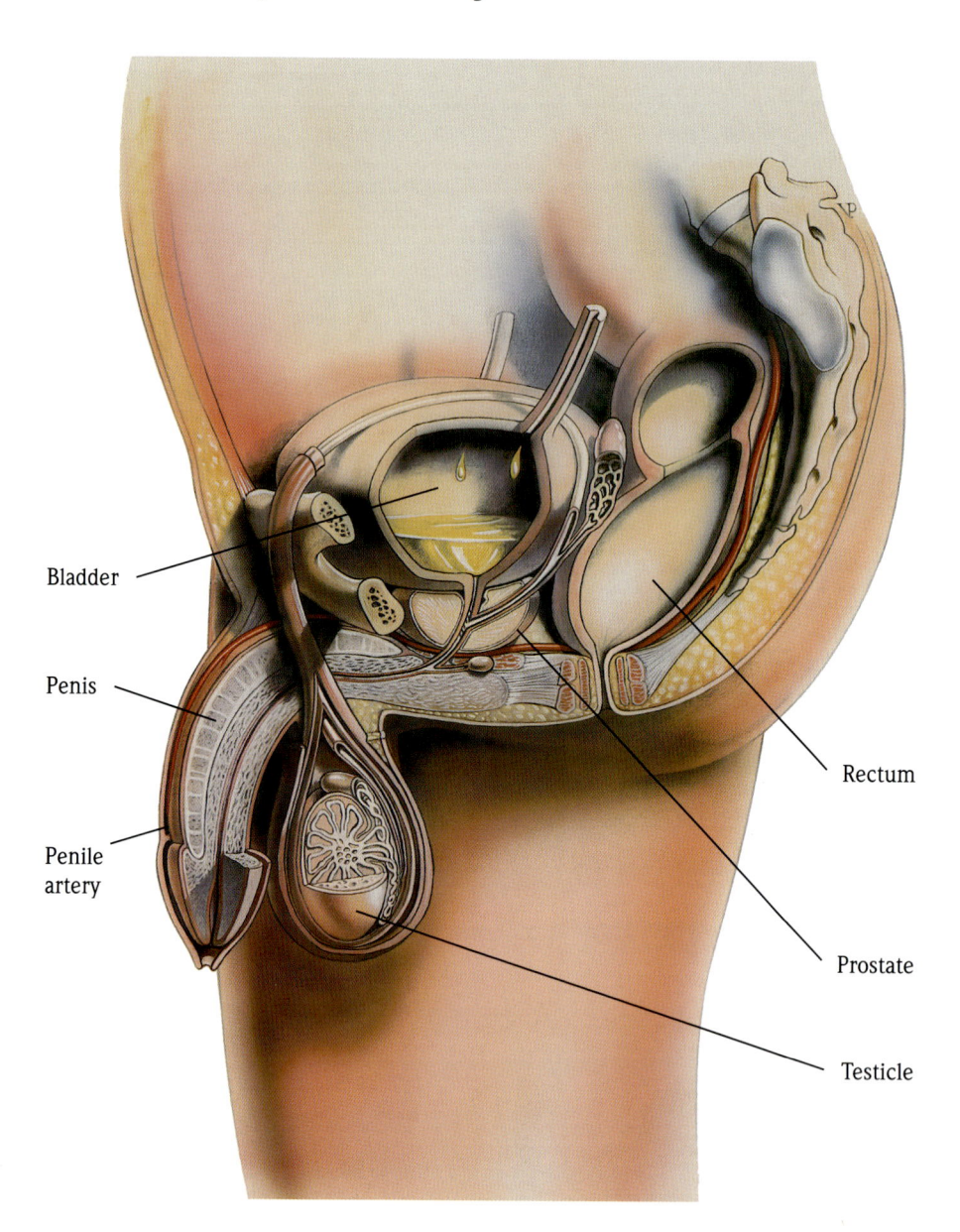

Testicle

During a rectal examination the physician will feel the prostate for evidence of a prostate tumor: enlargement of the prostate, excessive firmness, or lumps. The rather small penile artery is responsible for erections. Keeping it in good cariovasular condition and maintaining a satisfying sex life is dependent on the same healthy lifestyle as any other part of the body.

Osteoporotic Bone

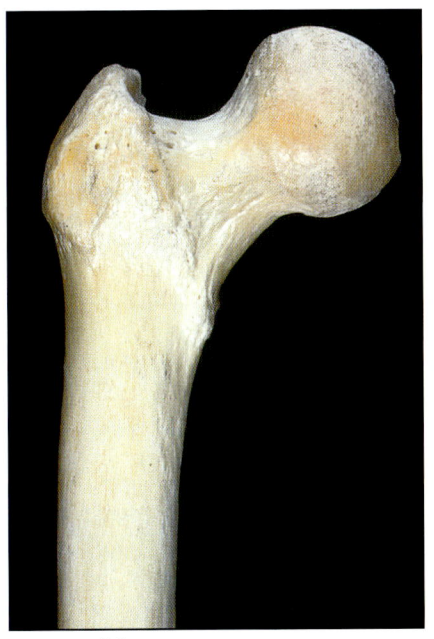

Plate 7

Healthy Femur

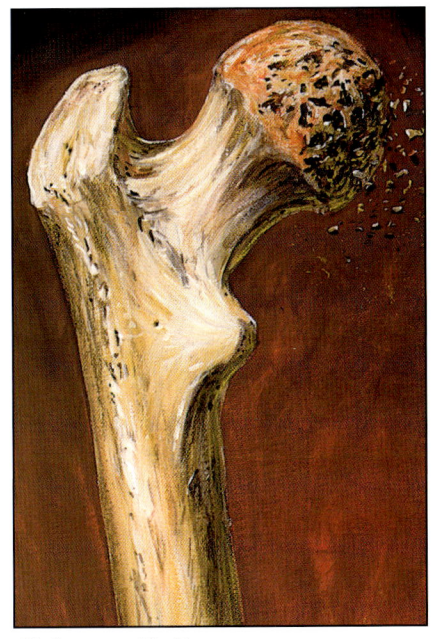

Osteoporotic Femur

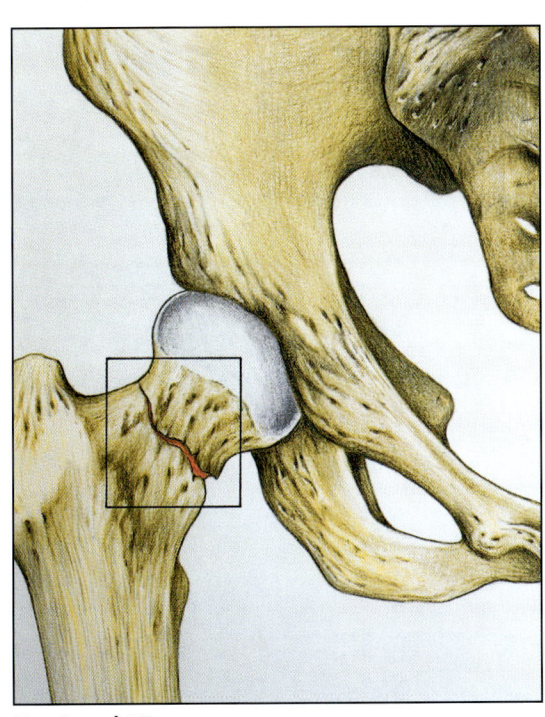

Fractured Hip

Osteoporosis can be caused by a sedentary lifestyle, smoking, and, in women, a lack of hormonal replacement therapy.

Skin Cancers

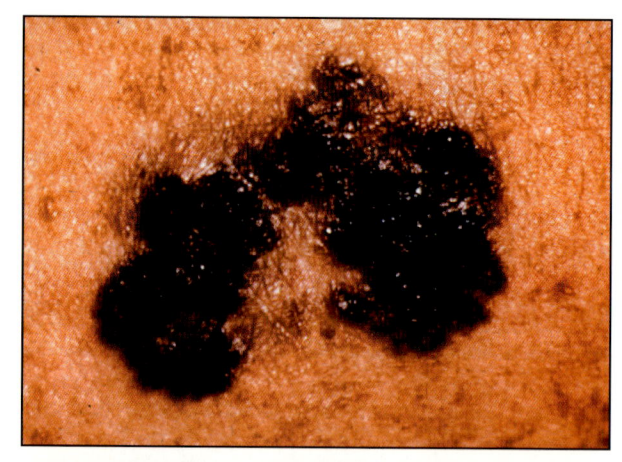

Plate 8

Melanoma: *The most aggressive and feared of skin cancers. Note the irregular border and variations in color.*

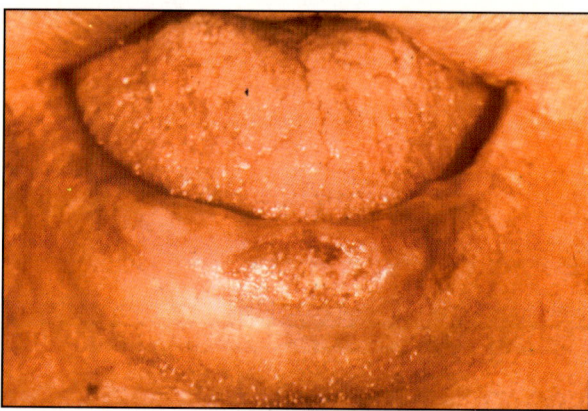

Squamous cell carcinoma *of the lip: Although less aggressive than melanomas, squamous cell carcinomas can, on occasion, be life threatening.*

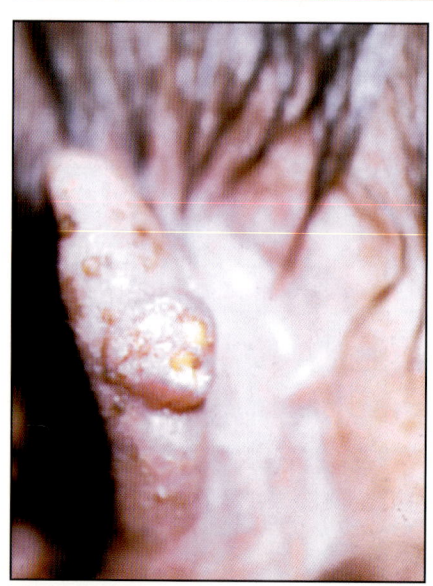

Squamous cell carcinoma *on the ear: Skin cancers are almost always related to sun exposure. All unusual skin lesions should be examined by a physician.*

Photos courtesy of University of Texas Health Science Center, Division of Dermatology.

SIDEBAR 12.1

The Antioxidant Revolution

Vitamin and mineral supplements have been around for many years, but only in the past two decades or so have we appreciated their use as *antioxidants,* thanks primarily to Dr. Kenneth Cooper, the physician who also popularized aerobics.

Antioxidants neutralize *free radicals,* which are atoms or molecules that are in an electronically unstable, highly reactive state. In the human body the most common free radical is oxygen. The evidence is strong that free radicals are a key factor in producing cancer, and, as a contributing factor in atherosclerosis, they also produce heart disease and other kinds of cardiovascular disease. Antioxidants act as chemical scavengers to remove the free radicals and thus retard the aging process. (Smoking decreases the blood level of antioxidants and thereby increases free radical production.) The best-known antioxidants are the vitamins A, C, and E and the mineral selenium.

The ideal way to maximize antioxidants is through a diet high in fruits, vegetables, and nuts. Antioxidants are so important, however, that I recommend vitamin supplements even for those who eat a superb diet.

Vitamin A is the antioxidant about which there is the most conflicting evidence and the most controversy. Several studies have shown lower mortality rates among those who eat foods high in vitamin A, but studies of those who take it in pill form have shown either no benefit or sometimes even *higher* mortality rates. Vitamin A in pill form should always be taken in the form of its chemical precursor, beta-carotene, which is converted slowly to vitamin A and is therefore known to be safer. However, even in the beta-carotene form, vitamin A has shown mixed results.

Some scientists believe that there are properties in vitamin A-rich foods other than the vitamin itself that account for the decreased mortality. Until the controversy is resolved to almost everyone's satisfaction, I believe that those who are convinced that the benefits of beta-carotene outweigh the risks should limit their intake to no more than 10,000 international units (IU) per day.

Vitamin C is known for reducing the risk of gastrointestinal-tract cancers, and it promotes wound healing and decreases the risk of cataracts. It has also been advanced as improving the immune system, especially by the Nobel Prize-winning chemist Linus Pauling. Unfortunately, vitamin C has also been shown to increase the risk of kidney stones, which, although almost never fatal, produce some of the worst pain known to medical science. I recommend taking 500 milligrams per day, which is unlikely to cause any such problem.

Vitamin E is the antioxidant about which I am most enthusiastic. It has been shown to reduce the risks of heart attacks and prostate cancer, and some researchers claim that it improves skin tone and increases "youthening." It has also been shown to alleviate the symptoms of PMS. I recommend taking 600 IU per day. Vitamin E is, however, a prohemorrhagic—that is, it thins the blood and promotes bleeding—and without a physician's advice it should not be taken by patients who are taking Coumadin.

Finally, the mineral selenium has been shown to reduce the inci-

---

A *randomized* study means that the patients are assigned to the treatment group or to the placebo group based on a coin flip. The reason is that if the patients or the doctors could choose between these two arms of the study, their choices might reflect biases between the two groups that would show up as different outcomes.

A *double-blind* study means that neither the patients nor the evaluators of the outcomes—usually the physicians—know which

dence of a number of cancers, especially gastrointestinal cancers and prostate cancer. I recommend taking 25 micrograms per day.

If it is really true that antioxidants reduce the risk of heart disease and cancer and, in general, promote longevity and youthfulness—and the evidence is strong—then the converse would be expected to be true: that one should avoid *oxidants,* or free-radical producers, the most controllable and avoidable of which is iron. There is, in fact, evidence that high blood iron levels correlate with some cancers. There is also evidence that people who donate blood frequently, and who thus tend to have lower iron levels, have far lower heart attack rates—although it is also true that blood donors are usually healthier than average for many other reasons.

Many women need iron supplements because of heavy menstrual losses, but postmenopausal women and men of any age almost never need them. Nevertheless, they are routinely included in most multivitamin preparations. With the new awareness of the potential hazards of iron supplements, it is now possible, with some hunting, to find multivitamin preparations that do *not* include iron. One has to wonder if all the Geritol sold on the Lawrence Welk show did more harm than good.

✤

patients are getting the treatment and which are getting the placebo; this is to guard against the placebo effect in the patients and against biases in the physicians. (An old joke in the medical profession is that a *triple*-blind study is one in which the researchers have lost the code, so nobody knows who got what!)

A *statistically significant* study means that there were enough patients in the study that the measured results, if any, were unlikely to have occurred by chance.

Finally, a *repeatable* study is one in which other researchers can perform the same kind of study and get at least approximately the same results every time.

Those are pretty tough standards. The truth is, though, that many health supplements are supported by anecdotal evidence only—meaning simply that somebody took the stuff and "felt better." That level of evidence is all but meaningless. It might indicate that further studies should be done to see if the stuff actually works, but it certainly isn't sufficient as a basis for someone in the medical profession to recommend the supplement as a treatment for a patient. And yet, some of the supplements that have received a lot of attention in the press have *never* been subjected to the kind of scrutiny I've just talked about. Notable for such lack of scientific validation are, for example, shark cartilage, and most herbal remedies.

Aspirin

Of all the health supplements that have been in the news recently, perhaps it is most appropriate to begin with the humble aspirin, a very old medicine that costs just pennies a day. Aspirin went into decline as newer drugs such as acetaminophen (Tylenol) and ibuprofen (Advil or Motrin) came into favor. Yet aspirin is now making a big-time comeback because of its ability to prevent heart attacks. There is also evidence that it is protective against colon cancer and that, like other anti-inflammatories such as ibuprofen, it may be protective against Alzheimer's disease.

The study that got the most ink was the Physicians' Health Study, which in 1982 divided 22,000 physicians into two groups, with one group taking an aspirin every other day and the other group taking a placebo. After five years of follow-up, the group that took aspirin had 44 percent fewer nonfatal heart attacks than the placebo group. For ethical reasons, the study was stopped early, and initially it seemed that everyone over the age of forty should be taking aspirin.

A closer look at the results, however, showed that, while aspirin undeniably reduced the incidence of heart attacks, it *increased* the incidence of hemorrhagic strokes, the most catastrophic type of stroke, caused by the rupture of a blood vessel in the brain rather than by a blood clot. The incidence of gastric and duodenal ulcers was also higher in the aspirin group—a risk that would be higher still in those who drink alcohol to excess or who smoke. (Anti-inflammatories in the ibuprofen class also produce higher rates of gastric ulcers.) Overall, there was no difference in the death rates between the two groups. Unfortunately, the study did not continue long enough to see differences in the rates of colon cancer or the decrease in the incidence of Alzheimer's disease that we would now predict with daily aspirin, based on the results of other studies.

I believe that the decision whether or not to take aspirin for people in their forties and beyond is actually a complex one. The argument for aspirin is stronger for people who are at substantial risk for heart attacks but at low risk for hemorrhagic strokes—specifically, for people with low blood pressure but other heart

> **SIDEBAR 12.2**
>
> ## Homocysteine and Heart Attacks
>
> Cholesterol levels have long been known to be associated with higher risk of heart attacks. Cholesterol is no less harmful now than it ever was, but an enormous amount of circumstantial evidence has linked high blood levels of homocysteine—one of the amino acids, the building blocks of proteins—with heart attack risk.
>
> Homocysteine levels, perhaps not surprisingly, are lowered by regular exercise and by a nonsmoking lifestyle. They are also lowered by adequate intake of the B vitamins B_{12}, B_6, and folate (also known as folic acid). Most of us who are not strict vegetarians will already be getting enough B_{12}. Vitamin B_6 is also easy to come by, since in the United States it is an additive in flour.
>
> Folate, however, is another story. A conservative dose of this B vitamin to lower homocysteine levels would be 400 micrograms per day. Those of us who eat foods rich in folate—beans, grains, fruits, and greens—will achieve that level, but those who are less zealous about their diet may not. It may therefore be wise to include folate

attack risks. There is also some evidence that a "baby aspirin" a day, or 81 milligrams instead of the usual 325 milligrams, will produce most of the decrease in heart attack rates while only minimally increasing the risk of hemorrhagic stroke. On the other hand, there are many people who should not be taking aspirin at all—specifically, those with a history of ulcers, those already taking the blood thinner Coumadin (warfarin), and, of course, those who are allergic to aspirin. On the whole, I believe that the evidence is strong for recommending a baby aspirin of 81 milligrams per day

The Evidence for Health Supplements

> in a well-chosen regimen of health supplements. This advice is doubly applicable to women of childbearing age, as folate dramatically reduces the risk of fetal defects that can result in spina bifida, a condition in which the vertebral column is malformed.
>
> The Food and Drug Administration recommended that all cereal-grain products be fortified with folate by January 1, 1999. Most breakfast cereals already contain folate, with a single serving typically containing 25 percent of the recommended daily allowance.
>
> In late-breaking news as this book was going to press, two new, and preliminary, studies showed a possible link between increased folate intake and decreased risk of colon cancer and Alzheimer's disease.
>
> The homocysteine theory of heart attacks and the likely decrease in incidence of colon cancer and Alzheimer's disease are not yet proven. However, the B vitamins carry little risk, the most important of which is peripheral nerve damage with very high doses of vitamin B_6. Adding these vitamins to the diet therefore falls into the category of "probably helps, unlikely to hurt."
>
> ❦

for both men and women who are over forty, have normal blood pressure, and have no special risks of bleeding.

Omega-3 Fatty Acids

Yet another older supplement that we have only recently come to appreciate is fish oil. Cold-water fish are rich in *omega-3 fatty acids,* a kind of polyunsaturated fat that remains fluid even at low temperatures. These substances are also found in linseed, flaxseed, soybean, and wheat-germ oils, and I recommend flaxseed oil (four 1,000-milligram capsules per day) for those who would like to supplement their diet with omega-3 fatty acids.

Interest in fish oils and their plant-oil cousins was sparked when it was noted that the Inuit of Greenland ate one of the highest fat diets in the world, consisting mostly of blubber-rich seals, while having one of the world's lowest heart attack rates. It was discovered that the cold-water fish oils they consumed were protective against heart attacks in ways unrelated to the lowering of cholesterol levels. The latter remain unchanged or, in some cases, actually increase in patients taking fish-oil supplements.

It appears that these unusually fluid oils in the bloodstream tend to prevent the buildup of cholesterol plaques in the coronary arteries. Further research demonstrated that the low heart attack rate of the Japanese, despite a higher smoking rate than that of Americans, may also be due in part to their diet, which is traditionally high in fish. (Ethnic Japanese in the United States eating our "traditional" diet of Big Macs don't get the same protection from heart attacks.)

These epidemiologic observations have since been confirmed in animal studies. There is also new evidence that omega-3 fatty acids may help to lower cancer rates by "crowding out" more dangerous types of fat molecules in human cells. Other claims made for omega-3 fatty acids, although with much less experimental evidence, include improved skin tone and relief from autoimmune diseases such as arthritis and multiple sclerosis.

Unfortunately, there is a cloud over these findings: omega-3 fatty acids are another prohemorrhagic, and the Greenland Inuit have among the highest rates of hemorrhagic stroke in the world. Again, it would be unwise, without consulting a physician, to start fish-oil supplementation if one is already taking Coumadin. While on the subject of hemorrhagic stroke, which can be devastating and which is, in fact, often immediately fatal, I am nervous that three of the health supplements for which there is the most evidence—aspirin, vitamin E, and fish oil—are all prohemorrhagics. I don't know of any studies showing the incidence of hemorrhagic stroke in patients taking all three, but I would be concerned.

Although it is hard to know the precise risk/benefit ratio for fish-oil supplements, I think it is safe to say that individuals who are not on a purely vegetarian diet will benefit from getting most of their protein from fish rather than red meat or chicken. However, inland freshwater fish such as catfish can be very high in mercury because of industrial pollution, and shellfish are in a different category altogether, as they are very high in cholesterol.

Garlic

There is probably no health supplement that has as long and distinguished a history as garlic. Garlic has been used as an antibiotic at least since the Greek physician Galen used it to treat the wounds of Roman gladiators. More recently, Louis Pasteur used it as an antibiotic, as did the physician and humanitarian Albert Schweitzer.

Among the benefits that have been claimed for garlic include antibacterial, antifungal, anticancer, antiatherosclerotic, cholesterol-lowering, free-radical-inhibiting, and antiaging properties. Unlike most other herbs and nonpatentable health supplements, garlic *is* supported by a body of scientific studies. Its antibiotic and antifungal uses are well documented, and in fact it was used extensively by American physicians to clean wounds during World War II. Among the other benefits claimed for it, the strongest evidence points to its effects in reducing atherosclerosis and inhibiting free radicals (see the sidebar "The Antioxidant Revolution"), in both cases probably resulting in a reduction in the risk of heart disease. Although further, and larger, studies of this plant would be welcomed, it can currently be considered to be in the "probably helps, can't hurt" category.

DHEA

Of several new supplements that have recently been in the news, DHEA (dehydroepiandrosterone) is among the more promising—and yet also among the potentially most dangerous. A chemical precursor of estrogen and testosterone, DHEA is produced in the adrenal glands at a rate that declines with age. There is some evidence that supplementing DHEA at moderate levels will increase energy, restore muscle tone, improve cognitive abilities, and enhance libido, although the studies that seemed to show this were *very* small. Similar types of therapies have been used for some time, with modest success, in restoring energy levels in patients with chronic fatigue syndrome, so there is good reason to think that those with normal energy levels might also find energy improved with this hormonal precursor. DHEA has also been shown to improve the life span in rats, but no such experimental evidence exists for humans.

In a recent study, Alzheimer's disease patients were found to have DHEA levels 48 percent lower than those of age-matched controls. Whether this is a cause or effect of Alzheimer's can only be determined with further studies.

Since testosterone supplements increase the risk of prostate cancer, and estrogen may slightly increase the risk of breast cancer, there is a theoretical risk that DHEA, which metabolizes to become both of these hormones, could increase the risk of one or both of these cancers. In Chapter 7 I talked a little about testosterone replacement to increase libido, a therapy that I believe is indicated only in rare circumstances, but testosterone has also been advanced as an antiaging therapy to build muscle mass and increase energy.

Given the known risks of testosterone, I would feel much more comfortable with oral DHEA supplementation in modest doses for those who felt that the benefits outweighed the risks of taking a supplement whose long-term side effects are not yet known. DHEA levels in the blood can also be increased in a more natural way through regular meditation, a finding demonstrated by the research physician Dr. Jay Glaser in 1986.

Melatonin

Hardly any health supplement has received more press recently than melatonin, a substance secreted by the pineal gland, a pea-sized body situated in the brain. Claims made for melatonin include better sleep and less jet lag, improved immune function, protection against stress and depression, decreased cholesterol levels, decreased rates of cancer and heart disease, and general youthfulness and rejuvenation.

Of these claims, only two are solid. Melatonin has been shown in human studies to improve sleep and protect against jet lag—results that are consistent with the natural fluctuations in its secretion (melatonin is secreted primarily at night). Unfortunately, all the other claims are based on animal studies, primarily in laboratory mice. It's unlikely that we'll see the kind of gold-standard human studies we talked about earlier, because melatonin is a naturally occurring substance not subject to patent. There is therefore no financial incentive for any drug company to develop and test it. Furthermore, much of the theorizing about melatonin is based on a view of the pineal gland as the "master gland"—an idea that is outside of mainstream medicine and for which there is no evidence.

The rationale for the use of melatonin, therefore—other than as a sleep aid—would have to be that the promising results in animal studies *may* extrapolate to humans and that it has no known risks or side effects. That doesn't mean, of course, that we won't discover any side effects. In fact, given the lack of controlled human studies and the short time melatonin has been used medically, it would be surprising if we did *not* discover side effects eventually. And since it is an unregulated drug, we have little assurance of purity in the preparations currently on the market, nor do we even know the proper dosage. Moreover, just as for human growth hormone and testosterone, there is a natural way to increase melatonin levels without taking oral supplements. Studies done recently at the University of Massachusetts Medical Center and the University of Western Ontario found that people who meditated regularly had even higher levels of melatonin than those who took the "usual" 5-milligram-per-day dose.

Human Growth Hormone

Finally, a few words about a supplement I would flatly discourage: human growth hormone. Growth hormone has been shown in some studies to increase muscle mass in men over sixty, while reducing body fat and cholesterol levels. However, other studies have failed to confirm these results, and the hormone is known to cause fluid retention and exacerbate diabetes. It also has the important "side effect" of poverty, costing at least a thousand dollars a month. There is a case to be made for all the other supplements discussed in this chapter—although with the caveat that in each case there are highly regarded experts who have looked at the same data and who argue against them—but I would discourage adult patients from taking growth hormone. If you'd like to boost your growth hormone levels, do it the same natural way that testosterone levels can be raised—through regular exercise.

❧ ❧ ❧

I have the sense that we are on the verge of an era of health supplements that will dramatically improve our health and longevity; however, I'm not convinced that we're there yet. Of all the supplements I've discussed, the only ones I believe beyond a doubt have benefits that outweigh their risks are vitamins C and E, garlic, and B-complex vitamins. Even then, it's possible to find knowledgeable physicians who will passionately argue the other way.

Above all, don't fall into the trap of thinking that, because you are taking a certain supplement, you can safely neglect the basics of good health. I have a colleague in my emergency medicine practice who has never been able to stop smoking and who, when faced with the obvious harmfulness of his behavior, rationalizes it by saying that he takes antioxidants every day. There are, unfortunately, no magic pills, and there's no substitute for the all-around health program presented in this book.

CHAPTER THIRTEEN

The Battle of the Bulge

Americans today live with a paradox about body weight. On the one hand, female models have never been so thin and waiflike, to the point that we are facing a crisis of anorexia and bulimia among female adolescents, while male idols, the adventurers ready to rock climb or mountain bike or even live out the James Bond fantasy, remain as fit and trim as ever.

On the other hand, *real* Americans have never been so overweight. About a third of our population is now seriously above ideal weight. Our society is aging as a result of medical advances and the declining birth rate, yet, even adjusting for our increasing average age, we have typically gained almost ten pounds in the past decade. Especially worrisome is the skyrocketing number of adolescents who are obese, leading some people to wonder if the demographic group that follows Generation X will come to be known as Generation XL.

Despite what seems on the surface to be a craze for fitness, only one in five Americans gets even twenty minutes of aerobic exercise three times a week—the bare minimum. Increasingly, we sit not just in front of the television all day, as we have done since the early 1950s, but also in front of the computer or the Internet terminal. We used to be bombarded with the temptation of junk food at the checkout counter; now it is not just the supermarket, but also the gas station with the built-in fast-food restaurant, or even the checkout counter at the office-supply superstore, that puts temptation within easy reach. And the trend toward "supersizing" in fast food "restaurants" has, not surprisingly, resulted in the supersizing of their customers.

Being overweight drains people of energy. Although those who are afflicted often resent the "weightism" of society, so much of our physical attractiveness is tied up in being slim that much of our self-esteem depends on our weight. Being overweight not only affects how attractive we are to our sex partner, but, at a certain point, a large girth can make achieving sexual intercourse almost impossible.

Although losing weight for medical reasons seems to be the least of the motivators for most people, there are legions of reasons why being overweight is damaging to our health. There is a close relationship between weight and blood pressure. Almost all Type 2 diabetics are overweight. Heart attacks are much more common in the overweight—although it is controversial how much of this risk is due to the weight itself and how much is due to the high blood pressure, high cholesterol, Type 2 diabetes, and lack of exercise that are so often found in the overweight. Varicose veins and hemorrhoids are also found more often in the overweight.

Almost all patients who have the *Pickwickian syndrome*—named after the Charles Dickens character—are seriously obese. Pickwickians snore at night and often fitfully wake up. Aside from feeling chronically fatigued (often leading to falling asleep at the wheel), they are at higher risk for heart attacks because of the sometimes dangerously low levels of oxygen in their blood during their disturbed sleep.

Blood clots in the legs and thighs, which can move into the lungs as pulmonary emboli, are much more common in the overweight. So are gallstones. In men, colon, rectal, and prostate cancers are more common. In women, uterine, breast, and ovarian cancers are more common. And women who are overweight are far more likely to be infertile.

In short, being overweight can kill you. Shakespeare's Henry IV was right to tell the corpulent Falstaff:

Make less thy body hence, and more thy grace;
Leave gormandising; know the grave doth gape
For thee thrice wider than for other men.

I wish I could write a chapter called "Losing Weight Made Easy" or "Melt Off Pounds While You Sleep." In truth, losing

> **SIDEBAR 13.1**
>
> ## 44% of Your Calories Come from This
>
> If you eat a typical American diet, 44 percent of all your calories come from animal products. As unappetizing as it sounds when we stop to think that we are eating our furry, feathered, and finned friends and their products, that's what our intake of meat, poultry, fish, eggs, milk, and cheese adds up to.
>
> Whether a strictly vegetarian diet is ideal is controversial, but there is no doubt that we can get all the protein and vitamins we need from a diet with 10 percent or less of animal products. We are far better off maximizing our intake of plant products: fruits, vegetables, grains, and nuts.
>
> Aside from animal products being high in fat and cholesterol and low in fiber, they are high in concentrated pesticides, which is probably why sperm counts have dropped by about 50 percent in the industrialized world during the last four decades. Animal products are also very low in the antioxidants that slow down aging and prevent cancer. Because plant products are so high in fiber and low in

weight and keeping it off are among the toughest health challenges, right up there with stopping smoking. I myself tend to run about fifteen pounds overweight, because of the ultrahigh stress of emergency room shifts, coupled with the easy availability of unhealthy, high-fat hospital food.

There is definitely a genetic component to being overweight. We know from studies of twins separated at birth that both will tend to run about the same weight, regardless of the environment they are in. There is no question that some people have slower

calories relative to their weight, people on a mostly vegetarian diet can eat far more without weight gain.

Those in long-lived societies, such as the Hunzas of Pakistan, eat an almost totally vegetarian diet. During World War II, when meat became unavailable in occupied Denmark and Norway, natural death rates plummeted.

To summarize:

	Animal Products	**Plant Products**
Fats	Very high	Very low
Cholesterol	Very high	Almost none
Calories	High	Low
Fiber	Almost none	Very high
Antioxidants	Low	High
Pesticides	Highly concentrated	Low (none in organic produce)

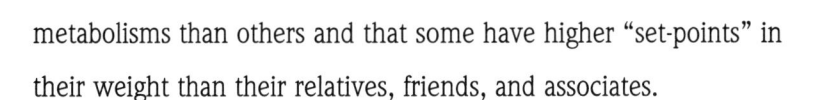

❧

metabolisms than others and that some have higher "set-points" in their weight than their relatives, friends, and associates.

Having acknowledged that, though, I would also have to say that many people who insist that they can't lose weight without drugs are, in fact, not yet doing all they need to do with diet and exercise. The plain facts are that the American diet is very high in fat and most Americans are very sedentary. Therefore, just doing more than your friends are doing does not necessarily mean that you are doing *enough.* Again and again I've had patients tell me,

"Diet and exercise don't work for me." When I question them closely, it often turns out that by "diet" they mean they've given up desserts, and by "exercise" they mean they are walking twenty minutes three times a week. In fact, what is needed to knock off the pounds and keep them off is not just giving up desserts, but eating a low-fat meal for the main course; and the kind of exercise needed is more like forty-five minutes of really vigorous exercise five times a week.

People sometimes say there is no point in exercising, because exercise just makes them hungry. Although the relationship between exercise and hunger is a complex one, exercise, in general, tends to *reduce* hunger. In one study, overweight women participated in a moderate exercise program for eight weeks. Even though there were no limits on how much they could eat, they lost an average of about fifteen pounds each.

With regard to the diet drugs physicians are often asked for, everyone probably already knows that Redux and (Pondimin) fenfluramine (the latter half of the fen-phen combination) were pulled from the market by the Food and Drug Administration in 1997 because of the risk of heart-valve problems. Amphetamines have always had an extremely questionable risk/benefit ratio for weight loss. And, while there might be an argument for using thyroid drugs to bring patients up to the high end of normal on thyroid tests, going beyond that point is just bad medicine.

What that leaves us with is Prozac, which has been shown to be helpful in weight loss with minimal risk, and a new drug called

Meridia (sibutramine), which has been demonstrated to work in reducing weight, but at a cost, in many patients, of higher blood pressure—a problem most overweight people have even without taking a medication that worsens it. Meridia is also a controlled substance, as patients can become habituated to it and develop cravings for the drug.

There is also another new weight-loss drug named Xenical (orlistat), which was approved by the FDA in 1999. It acts at the intestinal level by preventing the absorption of about 30 percent of dietary fat. It results in the side effects of oily stools and flatus (the polite term for passing gas). The use of Xenical was associated with a higher rate of breast cancer in clinical trials. Given the way it works, that association was probably due to chance, but we won't know for sure until we have several more years of experience with this new drug on a wide scale.

At least as important to weight loss as exercise, and possibly drugs, is the emotional component. For many of us, eating is a substitute for emotional closeness or for security when we are anxious or stressed. There is a strong correlation between eating disorders and childhood or adolescent sexual abuse in women, including the other side of the coin of overeating: anorexia and bulimia. I suspect that there would be the same correlation in men if boys and male adolescents were sexually abused at the same rate as females.

Even aside from the extremes of outright eating disorders, however, food plays a fundamental role in the psychic theater of all of

SIDEBAR 13.2

21 Ways to Lose 21 Pounds

1. Drink at least five glasses of water a day. A good deal of what passes for hunger is really thirst, because most "solid" foods have a high water content. The extra water in your diet will help give you a "full" feeling. Tossing in some shaved ice will even give you something to munch on that has exactly zero calories.

2. Give yourself permission not to have to eat everything on your plate. Despite what your parents may have told you, cleaning your plate will not benefit children in the Third World.

3. Pay attention to other people's weight-loss success stories. Tell yourself that if they succeeded, you can too.

4. Switch your late-night snacks to early breakfasts. A good breakfast really is the key to good nutrition, and skipping breakfast is almost certainly counterproductive to weight loss.

5. Dilute fruit juices with water or zero-calorie soda.

6. Share desserts if you absolutely can't resist them.

7. Don't bring the food that is your biggest temptation into your house.

8. Go grocery shopping on a full stomach—it will help you make sensible choices.

9. Just as those who have trouble sleeping should use their bedroom only for sleeping (and sex), use your kitchen and dining room just for eating, and don't eat in other parts of the house. That way, you won't associate your living room with eating.

10. Remove the sweets you've squirreled away—especially those candy bars in your desk.

11. When the urge to eat strikes, wait five minutes before eating to see if it goes away. Much of what passes for hunger is habit.
12. Diet with a friend or as part of a group. You'll appreciate the support, and besides, it's a great way to meet other nice people.
13. Eat frequent small meals, rather than two or three large meals.
14. Be very clear to your friends and family about your weight-loss goals. If you're dieting, the last thing you need is someone bringing you a high-calorie treat and saying, "I made it just for you."
15. Go out dancing, miniature golfing, or just for a walk—*anything* active, especially if your usual "activity" revolves around the TV or the Internet.
16. If you use food as a reward, establish a new reward system. Give yourself more time for walking the dog instead of eating sweets. You *and* your dog will benefit.
17. If you plateau at a certain weight, don't panic. It's normal to plateau—often more than once—as you lose weight.
18. Keep plenty of low-calorie snack foods around the house, such as carrot sticks and air-popped popcorn, which is a great food: nutritious, filling, low in calories, and high in fiber.
19. Avoid high-fat snack foods that are easy to eat in large amounts without intending to.
20. Weigh yourself once a week at the same time, to avoid the discouragement of the normal ups and downs from day to day.
21. Above all, if you backslide, tell yourself you've lost a battle but *not* the war. Acknowledge the error, and then get back on the program.

us. As children, we learned at the kitchen table the fundamental lessons of hunger and satisfaction, of food as an expression of our mothers' love for us and of control and manipulation. As we grew older, for most of us the family meal was one of the most important sources of intimacy and bonding in our families. One of the key factors behind the weight gain of the typical American is that we are spending so much less time on the family meal, and we therefore use food as a substitute for the love and closeness that were once expressed at the dinner table.

As teenagers, we learned that offering food seemed to enhance our budding romantic relationships. In one study, when women were asked what stimulated them sexually, one of the most common—and surprising—replies was that they felt turned on when a potential sex partner offered them food. There seems to be a primordial evolutionary message in the offer of food from a man to a woman, an assurance that "I'll take good care of you if you'll be my mate." Later, the roles often reverse, and it is the wife who shows her love for her husband by cooking the family meal. These messages of food as love are not lost on us, and when emotional closeness is lacking, we often turn to food as a substitute.

Those who suspect that they have an emotional connection with food would be wise to confront it head-on. There are now both group therapies and individual psychotherapy available in cities of even moderate size for people with this problem. Of the two, group therapy appears to be more effective. Most of us who are dealing with psychological problems will benefit from the reassurance that we are truly not alone and from the mutual support of others in the same situation.

Some people may also benefit from participating in groups that are not necessarily just about weight loss. Almost any of the groups that are devoted to overall fitness are supportive of those who want to address using food as a substitute for affection. Involvement in a church group can be a wholesome and useful way to address our temptations; at the very least, it is much better than staying home alone and dealing with the awful knowledge that there is a gallon of ice cream in the freezer.

Perhaps because there *is* such an emotional overlay to eating, it is not surprising that so many people are yo-yo dieters—people who can restrict their food intake long enough to lose a substantial amount of weight, but who, upon approaching their goal, then unleash all the cravings they had held in check and gain back at least as much as they had lost. The bad news about yo-yo dieting is that the overall weight trend of these people is *upward:* Again and again, they tend to regain more weight than they lost through dieting.

As tough as it is to lose weight and *keep* it off, there are a few key commonalities among those who have done it. These suggest the following recommendations.

First, don't go it alone. We are all social animals, and we need the support and encouragement of other, like-minded people—especially our loved ones.

Second, when it comes to food and exercise, environment is stronger than will. Arrange to have only healthy, wholesome food in

> **SIDEBAR 13.3**
>
> ## Pumping Iron for Weight Maintenance
>
> Most people find that pumping iron (weight training) results in little weight loss, since the increase in muscle mass tends to counterbalance the loss of fat. It does, however, redistribute the weight in ways that are esthetically attractive and that enhance self-esteem.
>
> Furthermore, pumping iron helps to prevent weight gain through a little-understood physiological principle. A given weight of muscle is far more metabolically active, and therefore uses far more calories each day, than the same weight of fat. Thus, even with the same-calorie diet, converting some of your weight from fat to muscle will help you to maintain ideal weight and keep off the pounds you've lost.

the refrigerator or the cupboard. Schedule yourself for regular exercise in which you must be somewhere at a certain time, lest your friends or colleagues notice your absence. The aerobics classes that some large companies offer on the lunch hour or after work are ideal. So is living in one of the Club Med-style apartment complexes that have a swimming pool, a gym, and scheduled aerobics classes.

Third, eat only at designated mealtimes. Don't eat your breakfast in the car while driving to work or your take-out lunch while at your desk. There is just too much temptation to wolf down greasy fast food in those kinds of situations.

Fourth, eat a larger number of smaller meals that add up to the same number of calories. Eating five small meals a day totaling

> **SIDEBAR 13.4**
>
> ## The Worst Exercise for Losing Weight
>
> Swimming is a superb all-around exercise that provides excellent aerobic benefits and muscle strengthening with minimal stress to the joints. Unfortunately, however, there is emerging evidence that swimming only minimally promotes weight loss. It appears that submerging the human body in water that is below body temperature sends a signal to the brain to *add* to the fat layer, to guard against the cold. In the long run, this tends to counteract the benefits of burning calories through the physical exertion of swimming.
>
> Swimming may still have a place in weight loss, but it is probably best to include it in an overall exercise program along with other aerobic exercises, such as brisk walking, jogging, bicycling, or aerobics.

1,500 calories will result in greater weight loss than three meals adding up to the same number of calories or, worse still, two humongous meals. Disciplining yourself to this kind of controlled, sustainable diet will help you avoid yo-yo dieting.

Fifth, give up alcohol. I never cease to be amazed at how many people feel that their alcohol intake is not a part of their diet. Many people like to tell themselves that a drink or two is good for their heart, and while that may be true, it is very *bad* for the waist. Alcohol is sky-high in calories! Beer bellies are called that for good reason.

Finally, if you relapse, acknowledge the mistake and get back on the program. Backsliding only means you've lost a battle, not the war. Don't go off the program altogether because of a momentary weakness.

If there is one last thought I'd like to offer you, it is to go for the full makeover. I have nothing against losing five or ten pounds, but if you really need to lose forty, the five or ten won't make enough difference in the way you look or feel to give you the positive feedback you need. Go for it! Unplug the TV, turn off the Internet, trash the junk food, bicycle to work. There is a new, fitter, healthier, revitalized you waiting to be discovered.

CHAPTER FOURTEEN

How to Avoid Doing Yourself In ❧

If I picked any hospital at random and took you on a tour through it, what we would find as we did rounds on the patients together and leafed through their charts is that most of them were there because they did themselves in. Many diseases are not preventable, such as juvenile-onset (Type 1) diabetes or arthritis. However, far more of the ailments that plague us are self-inflicted, and chief among these are the many diseases caused by tobacco and alcohol.

Part of me wonders if talking about cigarettes and liquor in a book of this kind isn't preaching to the choir. One would like to think that avoiding these obvious hazards would be most people's first step on the road to ideal health, yet I know this isn't true. From my years of practice, I realize there are thousands of good, well-meaning people who recognize that these addictions are dangerous but who have not yet been able to master the enemy within.

One would think that physicians themselves would be the most health-conscious of all people, yet the truth is that they have proved to be *more* vulnerable to addictions than the world at large. In the last two decades, the smoking rate of physicians has finally dropped below that of the general public, but their rates of drug addiction and alcoholism are still far higher than the norm. The drug addiction is presumably due to the stresses that go with the turf and the ready availability of drugs—chiefly Demerol (meperidine), an injectable narcotic that is a close relative of morphine and heroin and that is known sardonically in the medical profession as "vitamin D." The alcoholism is due not just to the stress, but also to the sense of isolation many physicians feel about the sometimes agonizing, and often lonely, decisions they must make. I'll always remember the time I was working at a remote emergency room where I was not one of the regular doctors, and telling an alcoholic patient what great people he would find in Alcoholics Anonymous. His startling reply: "Oh, yeah, I know, most of the doctors in town are in it."

Now, if physicians themselves—who have dedicated their lives to helping people with their health problems—are that vulnerable to addictions, it stands to reason that there are many health-conscious lay people who are fighting their *own* battles with addictions. Nor are these addictions by any means limited to alcohol and cigarettes; narcotics and cocaine also figure prominently. The truth is that modern society is marked by a great many addictive behaviors that numb us to the disappointments in our lives: food addictions (including the opposites of pathological overeating: anorexia and bulimia); gambling; the Internet; solitary electronic games; emotionally disengaged and joyless sex; and workaholism, my own constant temptation. Most of these behaviors in moderation have their place; an occasional drink with friends is hardly a danger to health, for example, and hard work can be a source of enormous satisfaction, as long as we don't allow it to rob us of adequate time for other vital activities in our lives.

What links these various addictions is that they let us push aside the things we don't want to think about and to avoid feeling the emotions we don't want to experience: the feelings of isolation, of inadequacy, of lack of fulfillment, of meaninglessness. Alcoholism also undeniably has a genetic component—it runs in families. And while loneliness often pushes people in the direction of liquor, alcohol is so damaging to our ability to carry on stable relationships that it is a *cause* of loneliness as well as a product of it.

Tobacco

Cigarettes are exceptional compared to most other addictions, because smokers almost invariably start as teenagers, when they have no concept that they are mortal or even that they will age. Teenagers start smoking for reasons that at the time are hardly pathological: a desire for social acceptance, to be "cool" or sexy, or

SIDEBAR 14.1

Health Effects of Smoking (Partial List)

Smokers carry twenty times the risk of lung cancer, more than twice the risk of heart attacks, and almost twice the risk of stroke as nonsmokers. Almost every cancer is far more common in smokers, and emphysema is virtually unknown in nonsmokers. Asthmatics will need medical care in the emergency room at least three times more often if they smoke. Male smokers are at three times the risk of impotence as nonsmokers because of damage to the penile artery, and their sperm counts are lower, making it harder for smoking couples to conceive.

Some of the chemicals in the witch's brew of cigarette smoke cause depression, which accounts for the higher rate of suicide among smokers than nonsmokers.

Smokers have more than double the risk of macular degeneration, one of the most common causes of vision loss. The fetuses of pregnant women who smoke get 25 percent less oxygen, resulting in more low-birth-weight babies and more premature deliveries. In later years, women who smoke will develop osteoporosis at twice the rate of nonsmokers. Women who smoke begin menopause an average of two years earlier than nonsmokers.

Passive smoke exposure kills many thousands of people each year from lung cancer and heart disease, and the children of smokers will get far more upper-respiratory-tract infections and ear infections, not to mention the damage from the bad example being set. Smoking impairs both the sense of smell and the sense of taste. Both men and women become physically less attractive because of more wrinkles, yellow teeth, and bad breath.

Smoking also causes the "side effect" of poverty: The average American smoker forks over between $1500 and $2000 per year to the cigarette companies for the privilege of being made sick or even killed.

out of a sense of rebellion—perfectly normal and appropriate motivations at that age. The problem is that nicotine is the most addictive substance in our society, and it later becomes extremely difficult to quit. Most smokers, by the time they reach their mid-twenties, have *tried* to quit, and there are countless intelligent, otherwise highly successful adults who, to their chagrin, are still smokers. My favorite example is William Bennett, author of *The Book of Virtues,* who, at the time he was appointed "Drug Czar" by Ronald Reagan, was still smoking!

It's pretty hard to reach adulthood without realizing that cigarettes are extremely bad for your health. However, I see over and over again that smokers consistently underestimate how bad their addiction is, and I get frustrated with politicians who say we should concentrate on the "real" drug problems of heroin and cocaine, when in fact cigarettes are a whole lot *worse.* Stopping smoking takes some serious motivation, and I think the first step is confronting just what a massive threat to your health cigarettes really are.

Cigarettes kill more than 400,000 Americans every year—about the same number that were killed in all of World War II, and far more than the number who die each year as a result of heroin overdoses, AIDS, murders, suicides, and car crashes combined. The Vietnam War Memorial in Washington, D.C. has the names of over 58,000 servicemen and women who died during that decade-long war carved in its black stone; about *seven times* that number die in the United States *every year* from cigarettes. While cigars are not as lethal as cigarettes, they are still extremely dangerous and can result in some horribly disfiguring mouth cancers.

Obviously, if you're reading this book you care about your health, and if you're a smoker, you've undoubtedly tried to quit many times already; the average adult smoker has tried at least ten times. Despite the criminal misrepresentations of cigarette pushers, nicotine is one of the most addictive substances known, far more addictive than heroin. And it is that rarity among drugs, a substance that is both a stimulant and a sedative. To the abundant experimental evidence of nicotine's addictiveness I can add my own experience: I've worked many times with heroin addicts in county hospitals, most of whom were also smokers, and *every one* who was able to kick heroin told me that it was much easier than stopping smoking.

To maximize your chances of quitting for good, you first need to ask for support from your family and friends. If you're married to a smoker, it's much easier to quit if you form a mutual support team; it's much harder if you're always around the cigarettes of your spouse. (Even if you can't get your spouse or significant other to join you, don't use that as an excuse not to do whatever it takes to quit.) You must lay it out as well to the rest of your family and your friends that you *need* their support. The sad fact is that some of your friends who smoke will feel diminished if you can give it up and they can't, and they may unconsciously try to sabotage your success. You must be very clear that you are serious about quitting and that you want and need their support.

SIDEBAR 14.2

Zyban for Smoking Cessation

Since 1997 there has been a very welcome new drug in the medical armamentarium to help stop smoking: Zyban (bupropion). Nicotine replacements, in the form of either skin patches or chewing gum, have proved their worth, but this new drug works in a completely different way, by decreasing the craving to smoke at the brain level.

Zyban is taken in pill form twice a day. It is a new formulation of an older antidepressant medication that was found more recently to be useful in stopping smoking. In one recent study, it doubled the smoking quit rates compared to taking a placebo pill. Perhaps best of all, it is completely compatible with the older nicotine patches and chewing gum, as well as the newer nicotine delivery system of plastic "cigarettes," which give those trying to stop smoking something to do with their hands. It was also found that smokers who used both Zyban and nicotine delivery systems had the highest quit rates of all, with a little more than half succeeding in giving up smoking.

One of the regrettable consequences of stopping smoking is that longtime smokers who quit often gain weight, typically five to ten pounds. Zyban, however, seems to decrease the tendency to gain weight.

The main side effects of Zyban have been anxiety and insomnia. It can also predispose users to seizures, so patients who have had previous seizures should probably not use this drug.

Part of your social support system should also include a smoking cessation group and the encouragement of your medical practitioner.

Some people simply get a flash one day that it's time to quit. They snuff out that last cigarette and never touch another. It's great if that works for you, but if not, try what seems to work for many people: Set a date that's significant for you—a birthday, perhaps— or set a date that's significant to both you *and* your partner, perhaps your anniversary. Put your reputation on the line by announcing the quit date to the world, and then, when the day comes, do what it takes to stick to it.

It's also entirely reasonable to try to cut down little by little, and then one day to stop entirely. Everyone is different—do what works for you.

Your chances of quitting are optimized by nicotine patches or chewing gum, which replace the nicotine in the cigarettes and which have recently become nonprescription remedies. (Nicotine is not what causes lung cancer—it's the other witch's brew in the cigarettes that does that.) By allowing the nicotine to be slowly phased out over a period of three months or so, many people find that they can stop smoking entirely. In fact, the nicotine patches or gum double the quit rate.

You might find it helpful to write out an affirmation, such as, "I am choosing an oxygen-rich body and a longer, healthier life. I am bigger than my cravings. I will succeed!" Repeat this out loud every time you crave a cigarette, and remind yourself that you are fight-

How to Avoid Doing Yourself In

ing a life-and-death battle, for the sake of your loved ones as well as for yourself.

Allow yourself, as well, some righteous anger at what the cigarette companies are doing to you. Remind yourself that they are extorting from you $1500 to $2000 a year to make you sick or even kill you, and then adding insult to injury by lying to you about the addictiveness of their product. (Not to mention their vile, cynical efforts to hook your children.)

Once you've stopped, though, you aren't over the hump—cigarettes are addictive enough that even as much as a year after stopping many people still feel a craving for them, which can be especially hard to resist during periods of stress. Therefore, to be a successful long-term quitter, *you need to find new ways to deal with your stress*—by exercising, for example, or by reaching for a carrot or celery stick when you feel that craving for something in your mouth.

If you do relapse, tell yourself that you've lost the battle but not the war. Don't use your setback as an excuse to stop trying. Throw out what's left of the pack of cigarettes, and get back on the program.

The day will come when you can pat yourself on the back and acknowledge yourself for having truly succeeded. You'll notice that you have more energy, that you don't get winded as quickly while exercising, and that you can smell and taste things you'd almost forgotten existed. The smell of cigarettes will only make you turn away in disgust. You'll feel great, and you'll never want to go back to the old you. And the really good news is that within five years or so, you'll be close to the risk levels for heart disease and lung cancer of someone who never smoked.

Alcohol

Alcohol is not nearly as chemically addictive as nicotine, but the insidious dependency that it creates is a downward spiral that invariably destroys the life of an alcoholic if not overcome. There are an estimated fifteen million alcoholics in the United States. Since confirmed alcoholism is rare before the midteens, that means that almost one American adult in ten has an alcohol problem. All of us know alcoholics, even if we ourselves might not have a drinking problem. What makes the syndrome less visible than it might otherwise be is that there is so much denial by its victims. While very few cigarette smokers deny being hooked, there are legions of alcoholics who could "stop drinking any time I wanted to."

Although the stereotype of the alcoholic may be the skid-row bum, many otherwise high-functioning people suffer from alcoholism, a disease that ultimately totally dominates one's life. The first step to recovery is to acknowledge the problem; a few simple questions, and honest answers, will help. Have you ever tried, unsuccessfully, to cut down on your drinking? When others confront you about your drinking habits, do you become angry and defensive? Do you ever feel guilty about how much you drink? Do you ever use liquor to get you going in the morning? Has alcohol ever damaged your financial stability or your marriage or friendships? Have you ever been arrested for driving under the influence? Do you come from a family of heavy drinkers?

All alcoholics need a social support system to stay dry. A thousand times I've heard the refrain, "Don't worry, Doc, I can handle this thing myself." It never works, though, precisely because one of the roots of alcoholism is a sense of loneliness and isolation.

That social support system almost always means Alcoholics Anonymous. Alcoholics Anonymous is a twelve-step program, and the first step is to acknowledge the truth. That's why, at the beginning of an AA meeting, all present introduce themselves by saying, "My name is so-and-so and I am an alcoholic." There is a crucial self-confrontation in that honest admission that is absolutely essential to progress. It is a godsend when an alcoholic takes that first step, and far more important than anything we can do in the clinic or the emergency room.

A second crucial step is calling on a higher power for help. If you're an alcoholic, I urge you to take that step. The higher power, as you understand it, might be God, or simply nature, or the universal energy force of the universe, or whatever you want to call it. The critical point is the acknowledgment that at this stage in your life, it is the liquor that is controlling you, not the other way around, and you need to draw on the strength of a higher order in order to prevail.

I've attended many AA meetings, and the fellowship and honesty I've seen have often brought tears to my eyes. On occasion

> **SIDEBAR 14.3**
>
> ## Health Effects of Alcohol (Partial List)
>
> Alcohol produces a profound alteration in one's consciousness—even when not actively inebriated—that leads to denial. This denial can persist even in the face of a cirrhosis of the liver that leads to *ascites,* or the taking on of fluid in the abdomen and around the ankles, and, in time, to the *caput medusae* (literally, "head of snakes")—disfiguring veins on the surface of the abdomen that are the body's attempt to circumvent this vascular failure. The liver failure, in turn, causes the blood ammonia of the victim to rise to the point that profound confusion and disorientation at the brain level result, often leading to outright coma. And pancreatitis is many times more common among alcoholics.
>
> Alcohol is one of the leading causes of congestive heart failure, in which the heart weakens and the lungs and ankles fill with fluid. Alcoholism causes stomach ulcers and erosions of the gut, which, combined with the bleeding problems typical of alcoholics, can cause hemorrhage beyond what can be stopped medically. Sadly, I've all too often held the hands of alcoholics as they bled to death internally after we had done everything we could to stop the bleeding and failed.
>
> Cancers of the esophagus and stomach are far more common in alcoholics. Alcoholism wrecks men's sex lives by causing both a

I have even secretly wished that I had some excuse to join AA, even though I've never been a drinker. Many alcoholics remain in AA long after they've gone dry for good, because the closeness and intimacy of the program keep them coming back and because they get deep satisfaction from helping others who still need to walk that road. There are some wonderful people in Alcoholics Anony-

testicular atrophy and a neuropathy, or damage to the nervous system, that makes erections difficult or impossible. And in women, this neuropathy dramatically decreases the ability to achieve orgasm. Alcoholism can cause a profound depression; alcoholics die far more often than nondrinkers from suicide, not to mention car accidents.

Alcoholism is the most frequent cause of *Dupuytren's contractures*, a disfiguring involuntary clenching of the fist that usually cannot be corrected without surgery. It also causes *spider angiomas,* vascular lesions that are most noticeable on the face. Because of the high caloric content of alcohol, many alcoholics are overweight.

Alcohol withdrawal, in its extreme, can produce *delirium tremens,* in which the patient shakes uncontrollably, experiences delusions such as insects climbing the walls and voices coming from the IV pole, and sometimes even has seizures.

Alcohol impairs social skills, and alcoholics lose spouses, family, and friends. Most alcoholics develop tremors, and their loss of memory leads them first to lies and then to outright confabulation, in which they invent a memory of the past to cover up for what they can no longer retrieve. Ultimately, alcohol pickles the brain, and at that point there is almost no hope, because the will to stop drinking is gone.

❦

mous, and if liquor is your demon, I wish you'd stop deluding yourself and get your rear end down to a meeting.

To those who have alcoholics in their lives, I can empathize with you. After years of confronting alcoholics in my clinic and ER and often getting exactly nowhere, I think I have some sense of what it must be like to live with an alcoholic. The sad truth is that denial is so much a part of the lives of many of them that they have to hit rock bottom before being able to look themselves in the mirror and acknowledge that they can't give up the bottle without help from others. I wish there were some other way to get through to alcoholics, but losing everything is sometimes what it takes.

If you do have an alcoholic in your life, ask yourself an extremely important question: "Am I playing a role in enabling this person to continue his or her alcoholism?" Codependency can often look a lot like helping, and if you find yourself making excuses for a loved one with an alcohol problem or some other addiction, you need to ask yourself if you have a payoff in continuing such a relationship. Sometimes tough love is the only kind that works, and sometimes the only message that will get through to alcoholics or drug addicts is to leave them. This may be exactly what *you* need to get your own life back on track, if you've done everything you can to help and still have come up empty-handed.

The children of alcoholics almost invariably have an especially difficult and lonely life, because many alcoholics are kind, loving people only when they're sober. When they drink, there can be a Jekyll-and-Hyde transformation that turns them into abusive monsters. A minority of alcoholics, on the other hand, are exactly the opposite: affectionate when drunk and mean-spirited when sober. Either way, the trauma inflicted on the children of alcoholics often lasts well into adulthood. Although people's reactions to growing up with an alcoholic parent are as individual as people themselves, many children of alcoholics find that they have an overdeveloped sense of responsibility. They often take care of others first, and feel guilty about standing up for themselves. They sometimes don't know *how* they feel or, if they do, have difficulty expressing their feelings. There are now many organizations and support groups for the offspring of alcoholics—both those who are children still at home and those who are now adults. If this circumstance applies to you, I urge you to seek out one of these organizations and find out for yourself how many people have undergone experiences similar to yours.

Now let's talk about the *good* side of alcohol. It has been demonstrated scientifically that a single drink a day is cardioprotective, that is, it decreases the risk of heart attacks. Not too long ago, data were released that seemed to show that the French had far fewer heart attacks than Americans, even though they eat a higher-fat diet and smoke more. The presumption was that this was due to the French custom of having a glass of wine with dinner.

It is true that a glass of wine a day is good for your heart. The problem, though, is that it's such a slippery slope. Two drinks a day is clearly bad and three drinks a day is a disaster. Aside from the issue of cardiac health, we know that even two drinks a day—an amount many nonalcoholics drink—decrease cognitive ability and predispose to Alzheimer's disease. And there's so much denial among alcoholics that these new data regarding alcohol and the heart have been agonizing to many physicians. The reason is that, while we don't want to conceal the truth, there is such a potential

> **SIDEBAR 14.4**
>
> ## ReVia for Alcoholism
>
> Until recently, the only medication for treating alcoholism was Antabuse (disulfiram), which makes the user very sick if alcohol is consumed while taking it. The improvement in staying sober is a modest one, because patients who have both the willpower to take Antabuse and the willpower to refrain from drinking while using it are generally able to remain sober with *no* medication. Antabuse also carries the risk of causing a potentially fatal reaction if patients go off the wagon while taking it.
>
> A second worthwhile drug for alcoholism is now available: ReVia (naltrexone). In its generic form, this drug was used in the past mainly in emergency rooms to reverse the respiratory depression caused by narcotic drugs. It has more recently been found to help alcoholics in remaining sober.
>
> ReVia is taken in pill form once a day. In one study, it was shown to double the abstention rates. However, the manufacturer warns that the studies conducted have been of patients in alcohol treatment programs, and it is unclear what, if any, benefits are achieved from taking the drug outside of such a program.
>
> The main side effect has been gastrointestinal upset. ReVia is known to cause damage to the liver in high doses, although in the recommended dosage it appears to be safe. It should not be used by people who already have liver damage or by those who are currently using narcotics.

in this case for the data to support the denial of so many people with alcohol problems that most of us can't in good conscience encourage our patients to drink at all.

The French data also proved to be inaccurate on close examination. Almost half of all heart attacks are immediately fatal: The victim clutches his or her chest, falls to the ground, and dies. In the United States, such deaths are almost invariably listed as presumed myocardial infarctions, or heart attacks, even if an autopsy is not performed. In France, they are listed as *mort subite*—sudden death—which effectively gave the French a lower heart attack rate, until the data were closely analyzed. It's still clear, however, that a glass of wine a day helps to prevent heart attacks, but the benefit is nowhere near as great as it first seemed to be in the French experience—and it *certainly* won't cover up for the sins of smoking and a high-fat diet. Furthermore, the propensity of the French to have a drink with most meals has led to even higher alcoholism rates than our own already high rates.

Addictions take many forms, but the common, underlying theme is that they are all escapes from a sense of loneliness and meaninglessness. For that reason, it is rare to find addictions in isolation—most people with a dependency of some sort have more than one. Of all alcoholics, for example, about three in four are smokers, which is about three times the smoking rate of the population at large. I often mention to my alcoholic patients that the two founders of Alcoholics Anonymous—one of whom was a physician—both died of illnesses caused by smoking.

A sense of meaninglessness and loneliness affects all of us from time to time—even the most successful, most socially adept of us—but it is especially profound in those who suffer from addictions. It is the addictions that not only cover up and numb that loneliness, but can also force us to confront it. I have worked with many addicts who were dealing with a whole range of addictions, some of whom fought losing battles and some of whom went on to win their war against the enemy within. Among that group that emerged triumphant on the other side, what I've sometimes seen is the miracle of their recognition that the addiction was there for a purpose: to get them to confront what they had to do to transcend their circumstances. A patient of mine is named Ronnie, an ex-alcoholic who is still active in AA helping others who still need to walk that road. To this day I can see in my mind's eye the peace and serenity in Ronnie's face the moment he told me, "Every day I thank the Lord for the insight He gave me about how I was deluding myself about my alcoholism, and what my drinking taught me about myself and my need to be bigger than the circumstances of my life."

CHAPTER FIFTEEN

Choosing Your Health Care Provider ❦

F inding a good health care provider can be an exercise in frustration. Traditional medical schools teach about disease diagnosis and treatment, but hardly any emphasis is placed on prevention and wellness. To these very old problems are now added the new ones inherent in HMOs (health maintenance organizations), in which the financial incentive is to do as little as possible for the patients, and managed care plans, in which physicians may be under gag orders that prevent them from saying what is really on their minds and in which reorganizations can remove physicians from their patients just when they have gotten to know and trust one another.

To a certain extent, I'm going to get on the soapbox in this chapter, because I consider our current system of training physicians very problematic. That's not to say that there aren't a lot of highly competent, caring, communicative, prevention-minded physicians out there, but the problem is that physicians like that exist *in spite of,* not because of, their training.

Medical schools start the job by selecting for many of the wrong qualities in applicants. Most of the emphasis is on the applicant's grades in courses such as organic chemistry, which is rarely used by clinical physicians, and on the scores on the Medical College Admissions Test, which similarly tests a lot of peripheral material. All of this information confers at least some theoretical benefit, but it tends to crowd out training for crucial, everyday skills that all medical students need. With ten students starting the ordeal for each successful applicant who gains admission to a medical school, premed students are left with no choice but to become hypercompetitive bookworms. Some university premed chemistry courses are even notorious for the sabotage of laboratory experiments that some desperate students perpetrate to gain a competitive advantage.

Medical schools claim that they also look at applicants' personal attributes, but there is little truth to this image. Unlike applicants for jobs as airline pilots, Peace Corps volunteers, or FBI agents, there are no background checks for applicants to medical school.

Once in medical school, students are immersed in an environment in which the patient is considered a purely biological system; in American medical schools, the mind/body connection doesn't exist. Truly central and eminently practical matters are left by the wayside to make way for the rote memorization of data that are available in reference books. At my own medical school, for example, there was virtually no discussion of human sexuality, and almost none on the psychological changes of menopause, with the exception of a few words in pharmacology class on mood swings and hot flashes. And, as odd as it must seem to those outside the medical profession, internists almost never receive any training in alcohol counseling, pulmonologists are almost never instructed in smoking cessation, endocrinologists almost never learn how to get their diabetics to take their insulin and follow their diets, and ob-gyns are almost never taught how to teach breast-feeding.

Not only was there no lecture on the connection between what people eat and how they feel, but the eight hours of instruction on nutrition that we were given during the four years of medical school were taught by a depressed, overweight physiology instructor who openly admitted that he could see *no* link between diet and one's sense of well-being.

Nor is there any meaningful instruction on physician-patient relationships. I got all the way through both medical school and my internship without doing a *single* supervised patient interview—what is known in medical jargon as a "history and physical." Think of what this meant: four years of medical school without a word about how to put patients at ease, how to establish trust and confidentiality, or how to support patients in times of loss and help them to find inner strength.

If the teaching and role models provided by the "attendings" in medical school—the senior supervising physicians—can be problematic, more alarming still is the all-too-common use of residents or even first-year interns as "instructors," graduates fresh out of med school who themselves are trainees. The blind lead the blind.

The students also find themselves in a system in which they are defenseless against mistreatment. Not surprisingly, some learn to treat patients based on the way *they* were treated as medical students and residents.

Much has been written recently about the dangerous and dehumanizing thirty-six hour shifts that medical students and residents must endure for years. Unfortunately, that increased awareness has led to little meaningful change, and the recent harsh cutbacks in Medicare and Medicaid have put even more pressure on teaching hospitals to exploit their residents. Not only are inexperienced residents routinely called upon to make life-and-death decisions while exhausted, but also they live for years on candy bars, coffee, and no exercise or social life—and are then asked to advise patients about their health! The husband of one of my medical school classmates wrote an article for the April 1993 *Harper's* about his wife's residency, titled "Is This Any Way to Train a Doctor?" It is a real eye-opener for anyone who still has any illusions about physician training. Both among residents and senior physicians, impairment due to depression, burnout, and substance abuse are common, and suicide rates among physicians is far higher than in the general population.

I keep reading in magazines about how medical schools are addressing these issues, and that they are training a new generation

Choosing Your Health Care Provider

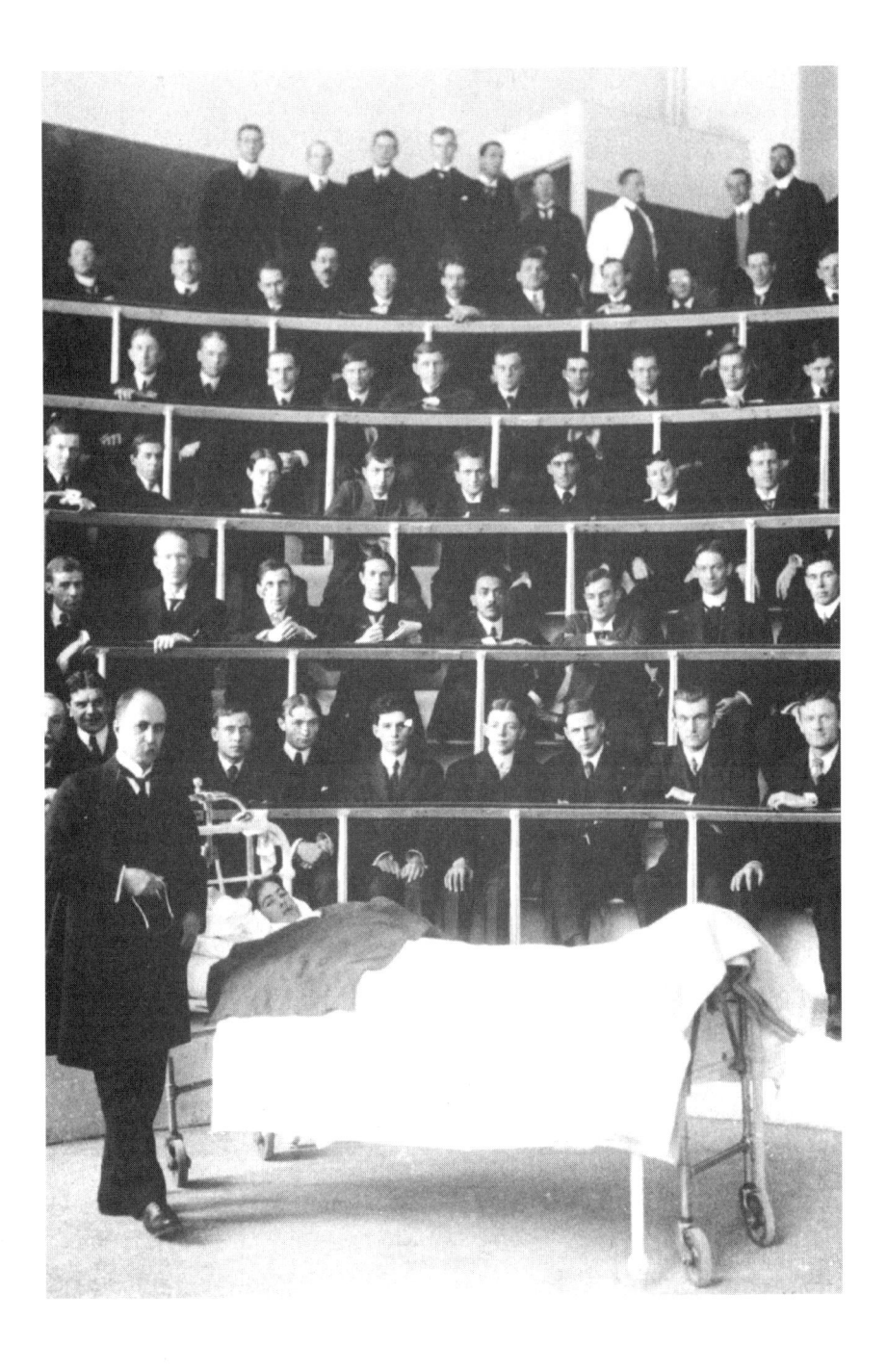

of physicians who are not just technically adept, but also able to bring the human touch to medicine. Frankly, I'm skeptical. Medicine is a government-protected monopoly; the number of medical schools and the number of openings for medical students have been deliberately limited to protect physician salaries. This policy has, among other things, left thousands of counties in the United States without a single physician. With three qualified applicants for each opening, and with no other source for the public to turn to for physician training other than the much smaller number of Doctor of Osteopathy schools, there is no feedback loop for medical schools and no incentive to change.

By the time I reached my residency, I yearned to treat the patient as a whole human being, and I chose carefully and well. In the family practice program at the McGill School of Medicine in Montreal, residents are supervised, with the patients' permission, from behind one-way mirrors by a senior physician or a psychologist who can observe four residents at a time. I'm convinced now that interviewing skills, or "bedside manner," can be taught, that active listening can be learned, and that the "playback" of what patients have said, to reassure them that they were truly understood, can be mastered. I believe as well that the connecting touch on the shoulder that has been known for centuries as the "laying on of hands" is a skill within the realm of even the less demonstrative student physicians.

The McGill program leaders videotape the residents' patient interactions. Thus was I able to watch myself miss the muttered expletive of a troubled patient that was the clue to his alcoholism—

a comment made while I was busy writing in the chart. Seeing myself as the patients saw me transformed everything I did as a physician.

The McGill program was also one of my first experiences of practicing medicine in a spiritual context. I was assigned to Montreal's Jewish General Hospital, where the patients were offered the opportunity of having rabbinical support to give meaning to the passages in their lives.

I held McGill in high regard, but a big part of the difference for me was that I was at last in a family practice environment. Family practitioners are only rarely found as medical school professors, because generalists are usually not welcome on medical school faculties.

In my ideal world, all patients would have a family practitioner. They are among the last physicians trained not just in the basics of all the disciplines of medicine, but also in seeing the human being within.

Family practitioners are among a tiny number of physicians who receive special training beyond medical school in psychiatry and the psychology of health care. The others are pediatricians, who study child psychiatry, and psychiatrists themselves, who rarely practice nonpsychiatric medicine. (On rare occasions, emergency physicians, the other true generalist discipline, receive some training in psychiatry.)

Family practitioners are a breed unto ourselves. We're not immune to the craziness that sometimes afflicts the medical profession, but as a group we are among the most people oriented and prevention oriented of physicians. There are bad family practitioners as well as good ones, but for a doctor who is willing to listen and see you as a whole person, and who can coordinate and advise you on any dealings you may need with specialists, a family practitioner is an excellent choice. (If this catches your interest, I recommend the book *Heirs of General Practice* by John McPhee.)

Unfortunately, there are not enough FPs to go around. In Canada, where I did my own training, about 55 percent of all physicians are FPs, roughly the same as in England and Australia. Most experts would consider this about the right percentage of generalists. In the United States, however, only about 12 percent of all doctors are FPs, while virtually every medical specialty is in oversupply.

Of the other disciplines that the over forty crowd might find of interest, internists receive broad training in the medical fields of cardiology, neurology, gastroenterology, pulmonology, nephrology, and endocrinology. They have more in-depth knowledge of these fields than FPs, but they don't have special training in gynecology, meaning that women who choose an internist as a primary care physician may need to look elsewhere for their yearly Pap and pelvic exams. Neither do they have special training in orthopedics, making them questionable for anyone who might need a physician proficient in sports medicine.

Many women these days get their primary care from an obstetrician-gynecologist, which makes a certain amount of sense, since the physician they spend the most time with will be the one delivering their babies and doing their yearly Pap and pelvic exams. Although ob-gyns have no postmedical school training in any field other than their own, they are generally well qualified in the areas that most women find of concern. Their motivation to do more primary care medicine may be due in part to the large oversupply of ob-gyns. Regardless of their motivations, however, many of them have become proficient in primary care, sometimes by taking courses aimed at preparing specialists to do more of the work of primary care physicians, of whom there are far too few.

In the title of this chapter, I deliberately didn't say "Choosing Your Physician," because I'm not convinced that physicians are always the best health care providers. One alternative to a physician is what has become known as "midlevel" providers—specifically, physician assistants (PAs) and family nurse practitioners (FNPs), who have become increasingly popular recently because of the great shortage of primary care physicians. These health care providers don't have the in-depth training that physicians have, but, on the other hand, their training is very focused on helping basically healthy people on an outpatient basis, and that might be perfect for you. Many PAs and FNPs are more humanistically oriented than the average physician, and, best of all, they often have more time than physicians do to sit down with patients and talk over what's going on. Most physicians have to divide their time between their inpatients and their clinic, whereas midlevels work exclusively in clinics.

I've found many alternative medical providers to be not only holistic in their approach, but also willing to devote much time and personal attention to their patients. One of the big downsides of having any kind of alternative provider as a primary health care provider, however, is that they can't prescribe medications, nor can they help women with their yearly Pap, pelvic, and breast exams. Even those patients who seek care from alternative medical providers will therefore find that they will still want to see a generalist physician as well.

Regardless of whether you choose a traditional physician, a midlevel practitioner, or an alternative health care provider, you are entitled to a medical healer with whom you feel comfortable and who has earned your confidence. If you walk out of the exam room not knowing what the diagnosis was, if you find your health care provider too busy or intimidating to ask questions of, or if you feel put down or demeaned by your provider, it is time to change.

Most of us have no control over the dysfunctional medical education system, but we *can* choose our health care provider, even if it means trying several before finding the right one. Study after study has shown that there is very little correlation between impressive credentials and either malpractice outcomes or patient satisfaction. What really counts in the long run is the thoroughness of the health care provider, the willingness to listen, and the honesty to admit that we in the medical field are as fallible as anyone else. Also very important are the empathy and compassion for patients that guide the healer to give them the same care that he or she would want in their place. Norman Cousins was right on the mark when he said, "Patients want to be listened to; they want to feel it makes a difference to the physician, a very big difference, whether they live or die. They want to feel they are in the physician's thoughts." If that's not the standard of care you're receiving, you have every right to walk out the door and not come back. *You* are in charge; it is *your* body and *your* life.

If there is one characteristic that stands out to me above all others as a predictor of the quality of care a healer can provide, it is the respect that he or she accords to the personal beliefs and outlook of the patient and to the dignity of that patient. On the Navajo Indian reservation in Arizona, where I did my basic family practice training, for years the Bureau of Indian Affairs tried to eliminate traditional Navajo medicine. The result was poor outcomes and an alienation of the Navajo people from Western medicine. More recently, after scientific studies showed that Navajos treated with both Western *and* traditional Navajo medicine did better than those treated with just one or the other, the official policy changed, and one of the newer BIA hospitals in Chinle, near Canyon de Chelly in the Four Corners country, has a permanent hogan adjoining it for the use of traditional medicine men.

Toward the end of my training, I had finally earned the trust of the Navajo people, to the point that I was invited to a traditional healing ceremony for a patient with pneumonia. The directions I was given took me through miles of open desert, and at each junction, I tried to follow the road that seemed to have more tire tracks. In time, I came upon several hundred Navajo people gathered under the vast sky, with several quite ancient medicine men surrounding the patient lying on a cot. Some of the medicine men were making sand paintings while others chanted a traditional healing song in Navajo as a wood fire crackled nearby:

> *With beauty before me, may I walk,*
> *With beauty behind me, may I walk,*
> *With beauty above me, may I walk,*
> *With beauty all around me, may I walk this earth,*
> *Wandering on a trail of beauty, may I walk.*

As I stood there, almost the only Anglo among a sea of *D'nai,* or Navajo people, under the warm early evening sun, I sensed the oneness the patient must have felt with the land, with the endless sky, and with the people of the Navajo nation there to support him. The understanding of how the potent healing of this powerful medicine of community and spiritual support would nurse him back to health—along with the antibiotics he was taking—became far more than just a dry scientific study, but an inner reality.

In the years since, I have often worked with nontraditional healing modalities, although I have to admit that, no longer having any contact with the Navajo people who were among my teachers, sand paintings and healing chants have not been among my resources. What I *have* learned, though, is the power of belief, the power of visualization. The patient's vision of the universe and of the healing arts is not just a consideration in choosing a modality, it is absolutely integral, and the physician who tries to impose the "right" medicine against the will of the patient is a fool.

The relationship between a medical healer and a patient is a sacred one, and the practice of medicine is not a job, but a calling. The ancient command of *primum non nocere* (first, do no harm), the covenant never to think of the patient in a sexual way, and the inviolable trust of doing what is right for the patient regardless of financial gain are as true now as they were two millennia ago.

CHAPTER SIXTEEN

If You Need Surgery

Most of us would do just about anything we could to avoid going under the surgeon's knife. While there are times when surgery *is* necessary, the basic message in this chapter reinforces the natural reluctance to submit to it. Surgery is an option to be avoided until every other reasonable approach has failed.

The good news is that, with very few exceptions, there is time to consider alternatives when surgery has been recommended. Appendicitis, strangulated hernias, intestinal obstructions, ruptured aortic aneurysms, and the like are true emergencies and can't wait, but most operations can be postponed to allow us to reflect and get a second opinion.

Surgeons, not surprisingly, have a bias toward surgery. Some of that comes from their training, but some of it is financial. A big part

> **SIDEBAR 16.1**
>
> ## Surgery for Angina and Coronary Artery Disease
>
> One of the most common operations in the United States today is *coronary bypass surgery*, in which one or more of the coronary arteries is replaced, while the patient is on a heart-lung machine, by either the saphenous vein in the leg or the internal mammary artery from the chest wall. The purpose of this operation is either to relieve angina caused by coronary arteries that are clogged with cholesterol plaques (see Plate 3) or to increase the pumping power of the heart in patients who have both clogged coronary arteries and congestive heart failure—meaning that the heart isn't pumping strongly enough to avoid fluid filling the lungs and ankles. A variant of this surgery is *angioplasty*, in which "balloons" are used to open up the clogged coronary arteries.
>
> These procedures are extremely risky. Bypass surgery carries a high enough mortality rate that it was only a few years ago, with improved surgical techniques, that it was demonstrated to increase anticipated life span. Bypass surgery typically lasts only ten years or so before a follow-up operation is needed. It also results in tiny clots being created during the operation. These clots travel to the brain, causing "mini-strokes" too small to appear on CT scans. Although most people feel as mentally sharp as ever following bypass surgery,

of the story, though, is that surgeons are a breed apart in their approach to medicine.

Surgery is a harsh mistress. Because of the vast amount of time surgeons spend in the operating room, in addition to seeing patients in clinics and hospitals, the demands on their time, both in training and as attending physicians, are even greater than the

studies have shown that the IQ of patients undergoing this procedure is lowered. Angioplasty probably carries less risk of the ministrokes, but it lasts a far shorter time, often requiring a new procedure to open the coronary arteries in only three years or less.

It is crucial for those contemplating bypass surgery to understand that there are tremendous differences in patient mortality rates among cardiac surgeons and among hospitals where this procedure is performed. A bypass is a *very* delicate operation and, aside from the experience, dexterity, and perfectionism of the surgeon, speed is of the essence. These operations are conducted while the patient's heart is *stopped,* and long operative times correlate with poor outcomes. There are some surgeons and some institutions that ought to be awarded black stars for their high mortality rates. Patients would be well advised to make in-depth inquiries about the reputations and mortality rates associated with the surgeons and hospitals they are considering.

The tragedy is that these operations would almost never be necessary if everyone followed the kind of program outlined in this book. Even for those who "need" such procedures, we now know from the work of Dr. Dean Ornish and others that these plaque buildups can be reversed with an aggressive enough health program (see Chapter 19).

❀

already daunting sacrifices required of nonsurgical specialists. Surgical training leaves almost no time to learn nonsurgical approaches; it's a rare orthopedic surgeon, for example, who has any mastery of nonsurgical therapies for back pain. Surgeons often don't have the time to sit down and explain the problem and the train of logic behind their recommendations, frequently leaving the task of explaining the surgery and its risks and benefits to generalists like myself. The results are interesting. A recent issue of the *New England Journal of Medicine* reported on a study of patients with chronic low-back pain, in which the patients reported the best pain relief after seeing a chiropractor and the second-best results with a family practitioner; orthopedists came in dead last.

A variety of elective surgeries are performed in the United States in numbers out of all proportion to their medical justification, and in *far* greater numbers than are performed in other advanced countries. Some, especially hysterectomies, as I noted in Chapter 9, are performed at vastly different rates in different parts of the United States, leading one to wonder if there is any science in how the recommendations are made. It is interesting to note that, unlike drugs, which must be demonstrated to be safe and effective before the Food and Drug Administration will license them, there is no such approval process for surgeries.

Operations for low-back pain, such as *laminectomies,* in which the posterior part of some of the vertebrae of the backbone are surgically removed, and *fusions,* in which adjoining vertebrae are rigidly attached to one another, are performed in much higher numbers than are justified by the scientific evidence supporting these surgeries, especially considering the great risks involved. Cesarean sections are also performed at greater rates than are justified. Cardiac bypass surgery, in which the diseased coronary arteries are replaced with an artery or vein graft, is performed at least 30 percent too often even by current standards, and would hardly

If You Need Surgery

be necessary at all if everyone would just follow the kind of preventive program outlined in this book. (Small voice in back of head: "Dream on, doctor.")

Not all surgeons are overly knife-happy, of course; at the moment I'm working with several surgeons who are veritable saints in the way they treat their patients and put their patients' welfare above any financial considerations. My bottom-line advice, though, is that if you get a recommendation for elective surgery, you should definitely get a second opinion, preferably from your primary health care provider.

If, after due consideration and a second opinion, you choose to undergo surgery, there are two crucial things you can do to speed your recovery. One, after clearing it with your physician, is to start taking megadoses of vitamin C of around 1,000 milligrams a day, which will speed the surgical healing by about a day. This is not news to any physician, but surgeons are so busy that they often forget to tell their patients. The second (and you don't need to clear this with anyone) is to stop smoking, if you are a smoker. This is the ideal time to do it. Smoking, because it attacks the arteries and veins and diminishes circulation, will dramatically slow wound healing, and it makes postoperative blood clots and pneumonia more likely.

You may be offered the choice between general anesthesia and epidural anesthesia, in which the anesthetic is injected into the space surrounding your spinal cord. If so, you are almost certainly better off with the epidural, as it is less risky, particularly with

SIDEBAR 16.2

Surgery for Back Pain

Those who suffer from chronic back pain will almost certainly be advised to have back surgery at some point. The three types of back operations most commonly performed in the United States are *disk surgeries*, in which a herniated disk is repaired; *fusions*, in which two or more vertebrae are joined, usually using a bone graft from the hip; and *laminectomies*, in which the portion of the vertebra behind the spinal cord is removed.

These surgeries are all highly risky, not only in terms of all that can go wrong during the operation itself, but also in terms of the long-term likelihood of scarring of the vertebral bodies that impinge on the nerves; such scarring will worsen the back pain rather than correct it. *Many* patients find they are *worse* off after undergoing these types of surgeries, which are performed far more often in the United States than in any other country. I strongly discourage my own patients from undergoing back surgery until they have explored every other avenue.

Back pain, along with colds and the flu, is among the most common illnesses bringing patients to see their doctors, and it is always tough to deal with. Among the first lines of defense is maintaining ideal weight, since being overweight tends to produce back pain all by itself. A high percentage of all back-pain patients are overweight, which can be a vicious circle, since exercise can be difficult while one is experiencing back pain. It is important, however, to remain physically active even while working through the back pain.

All back-pain patients who smoke need to stop, because smoking sharply increases the loss of calcium from the bones, and this causes osteoporosis, which will dramatically worsen back pain in time.

postoperative complications such as pneumonia and *atelectasis,* the partial infolding of the lungs. If watching the surgeon operating on you makes you nervous, the anesthesiologist can arrange a sterile curtain so you don't have to look. On the other hand, some people actually enjoy watching what is going on, and it will give you a chance to drive your surgeon batty by counting the sponges and making sure they all come out again.

During your recovery, once you've cleared it with your surgeon, it is important to start moving around as soon as possible. The old regimen of strict bed rest following surgery has been passé for at least twenty years; we now know that moderate exercise following surgery dramatically decreases the incidence of pneumonia, atelectasis, and blood clots in the legs and lungs.

Finally, I'll give you some advice you won't get from any surgeon. If you know you're going to need surgery, meditate regularly for a few weeks in advance. It will decrease your stress level, promote your wound healing, and decrease your complication rate.

Sound interesting? Read on.

CHAPTER SEVENTEEN

Meditation: It's Not What You Think

There is no question that people who derive meaning from their spiritual lives live longer and enjoy better physical and mental health than those who lack such an anchor in life. In the last few years, studies have piled up showing that, beyond any reasonable doubt, patients whose faith sustains them do better than those who are not on a spiritual path of some kind.

- In a study on patients with colorectal cancer in Melbourne, Australia, reported in England's *Journal of the Royal Society of Medicine*, it was found that those on a spiritual path were only about two-thirds as likely to get cancer as those who were not, and those on a spiritual path who *did* get cancer survived an average of ten months longer.

Sir William Osler
(1849-1919)

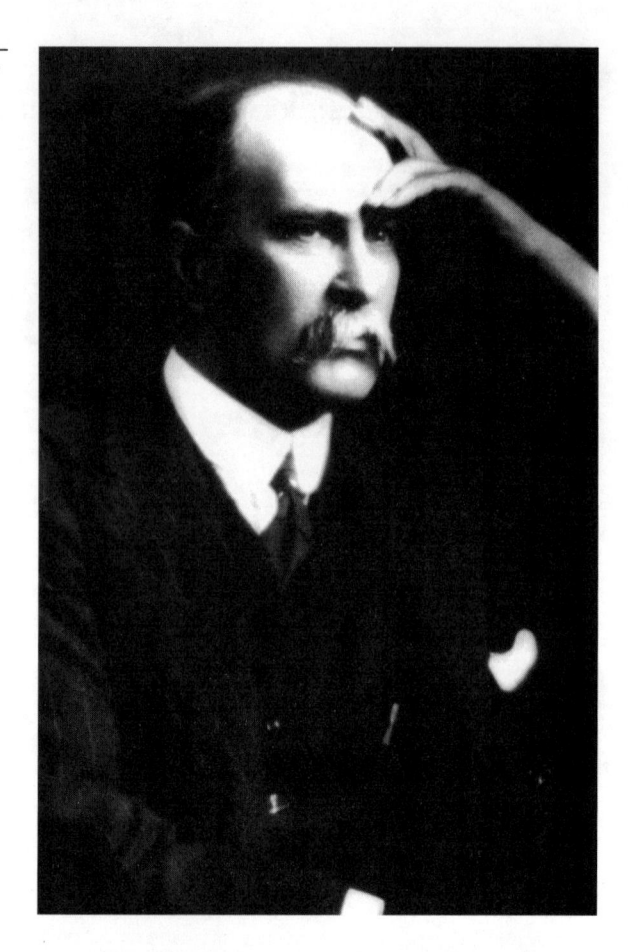

- A study by psychiatrist George Vaillant, reported in his book *The Natural History of Alcoholism,* demonstrated that those who entered an Alcoholics Anonymous program and trusted in a higher power were far more likely to attain sobriety than those who were treated through medical or psychological interventions.

- In a study done cooperatively by the University of Galveston Medical School and Dartmouth Medical School, researchers

Meditation: It's Not What You Think

found that those patients undergoing open-heart surgery who had no religious faith were three times as likely to die within the postoperative period as those who were not.

- It has even been demonstrated in one study that the patients whose physicians prayed for them did better than those whose physicians didn't pray. As Ecclesiastes tells us, "For of the most high cometh healing."

Sir William Osler (1849–1919), one of the founders of modern internal medicine and a professor at the McGill School of Medicine, is known as the one medical pioneer, other than perhaps the chemist Louis Pasteur, who most transformed medicine into a scientific practice in which experimental evidence proving the value of treatments offered to patients is demanded. So towering was this man's reputation that to this day there is scarcely a lecture hall at McGill that doesn't have a photo of him on the wall. I recall well, from my own years at McGill, taking inspiration from his countenance, a face that was at once serious and determined, yet kindly and compassionate. Such was his fame that the announcement that Osler would be visiting the wards with the residents and medical students stirred hope among even the sickest of patients.

It is often forgotten, however, that this giant of science was a deeply religious man (as was Pasteur) who very nearly chose the ministry over the medical profession. Even the most skeptical physicians of his day couldn't help noticing that, with seemingly nothing more than a reassuring hand on the shoulder and a few words of encouragement from Osler, even gravely ill patients sometimes made extraordinary recoveries and walked out of the hospital into the light of a new day.

Osler himself wrote,

Nothing in life is more wonderful than faith—the one great moving force which we can neither weigh in the balance nor test in the crucible. . . . Faith has always been an essential factor in the practice of medicine.

Phenomenal, even what could be called miraculous, cures are not very uncommon. Like others, I have had cases any one of which, under suitable conditions, could have been worthy of a shrine or made the germ of a pilgrimage.

The spiritual side of healing will always find a place in medicine, because spiritual strength is such a potent healer and because people have such a deep need to see meaning in the illnesses that befall them. I'm focusing on meditation in this chapter because it offers profound health benefits entirely aside from its spiritual dimension. It is possible to take advantage of the health and stress-reduction benefits of meditation with no expectation of any spiritual benefits—as I did for quite some time before the spiritual side of meditation stole into my life through the back door.

For those of you who are already meditators, I don't need to tell you about the benefits, because you know the heightened sense of well-being and the greater ability to deal with life's stresses that come through regular meditation, and you know how much you miss your daily meditation on those off days when things don't go as planned and you can't find the time.

For those of you who are *not* meditators, however, it is a notoriously difficult subject to address, because appearances are so deceiving and because meditation can be approached on various levels. Meditation is a vital part of the spiritual practices of many people. It also has some highly practical benefits to health, which can be scientifically documented. My own meditations began during an especially stressful period in my life, and I initially focused on stress reduction, which was immediate, deep, and out of all proportion to the time I invested in it. Eventually, however, the spiritual dimension of meditation crept up on me, and it is now by far the most important aspect of my meditations—although I can't say I'm unhappy about the effect it has had on my blood pressure.

What is difficult to communicate to the nonmeditator is just what meditation *is*. It often appears to nonmeditators to be a form of concentrated thought, when in fact it is precisely the opposite: a *stilling* of the mind. The classic double entendre of meditators is the bumper sticker "Meditation—it's not what you think." The difficulty in trying to express in words to a nonmeditator the essence of meditation is so challenging that meditation, perhaps more than any other discipline, embodies the ancient Zen proverb "When the student is ready, the teacher will appear."

Most of us, as we go through life, have an inner voice that provides us with a constant—and often repetitious—commentary: a string of judgments, regrets, expressions of wishes that things were different, and so forth. That voice has been termed the *Yama-Yama*. It is the purpose of meditation to *quiet* that voice to allow the realization of the true self—a process that, not surprisingly, is extremely difficult to express in words.

Although a friend of mine has written a book on how to meditate (John Novak, *How to Meditate*) even he agrees that it is far better to learn meditation from a longtime practitioner than to try to learn it via a "correspondence course," and I'm not going to describe the technique here. What I would like to do, though, is describe the enormous physiological and psychological benefits of regular meditation.

The quieting of the *Yama-Yama* through meditation accentuates the parasympathetic nervous system response which is the relaxation component of the nervous system that lowers the blood pressure, decreases the heart rate, promotes digestion, aids sleep, and is essential to sexual function, among many other effects. At the same time, meditation suppresses the sympathetic nervous system response, the fight-or-flight state that causes us to become nervous, sweaty, and aggressive.

Meditation has been scientifically shown to decrease the risk of heart attacks; decrease the frequency of irregular heart rhythms; decrease cholesterol levels; improve the functioning of the immune system; promote wound healing; improve tolerance for stress; decrease depression; decrease addictive behavior; decrease the rates of accidents, suicides, and homicides; and improve interpersonal relationships and sexuality. In 1978 the researcher Robert Keith Wallace demonstrated that regular meditators were physiologically *five to twelve years younger*—based on objective measurements of near-point vision, acuity of hearing, and blood pressure—than non-meditators of the same chronological age.

Regardless of the motivation for beginning meditation, its practitioners almost invariably find that it greatly deepens their spiritual life. I myself have had many moving spiritual experiences during my meditations that would be extremely difficult to put into words. If there is one discovery I've made that I *can* put into words, however, it is the realization that everything that happens in life is for a purpose and is a part of the great plan to teach us precisely what we need to know at that moment. As Richard D. Mann expressed it in *The Light of Consciousness,*

> *The body seems to be moved, purified; the imagery has an unfamiliar and awesome clarity; the spontaneous registry of what one's life and current experiences all imply at their core may take the form of searing insights. Even the stillness comes as a blessing and a discovery. Whatever happens, it continues to suggest a shift in the inner structure of one's consciousness.*

Like everyone else, I've had my share of life's tragedies, including a few that were deliberately inflicted by others and that at the time seemed utterly senseless. And yet, through meditation, I have sometimes had peak experiences giving me the insight that those tragedies occurred for a reason, that they had a purpose, and that I emerged stronger as a result of them. Meditation has given me an inner peace and strength that are difficult to describe.

The sense of oneness with others that is an almost universal experience of meditators grew on me, and in time I found that I could truly "get" that the experiences of my patients were universal. I came to realize that, but for the vagaries of a few different circumstances in life and a few genes that distinguished my patients from me, I could as well be them, and that in caring for them I was caring for myself. With some of the more unfortunate patients, I felt a deep sense of "There, but for the grace of God, go I."

My clinic days and emergency room shifts now begin with a prayer for my patients and a brief moment of meditation, and that has made all the difference. I suppose it is obvious that for an emergency room physician, life is stress, yet the meditation has made that stress tolerable. I believe that my prayer and meditation for my patients, my asking for my mind and my heart to be ready and for my hand to be guided, have served me in good stead.

The practice of meditation may be better known to the Eastern religions than to the Western, as is perhaps most tellingly expressed by Hermann Hesse in *Siddhartha,* when he said, "Within yourself there is a stillness to which you can retreat at any time and be yourself." Yet the principles of meditation are well known to Christianity. Perhaps the very essence of it is embodied in Psalms 46:10:

Be still, and know that I am God.

CHAPTER EIGHTEEN

When Things Go Wrong &

Having gotten this far in the book, by now you are probably feeling enthusiastic about the transformation you will see with these dramatic changes in your life, and are optimistically looking forward to making the years ahead of you the best ever. While there is no reason to doubt that those changes will occur, it is also true that at some point your ship will founder.

When we suffer loss, our attachment to the nonessential and the worldly is tested. When we lose our money, our belongings, our position, we are challenged to realize that what we have lost is *Maya,* the Hindu concept of delusion, of attachment to the fleeting and the material.

But when we lose our health—something we invariably take for granted until we don't have it anymore—it is harder to be detached. The realization that we can have serenity and fulfillment even with physical limitations doesn't come easily, and for some it doesn't come at all.

Some losses, though, test our ability to endure, to bear the unbearable, to suffer the insufferable. The death of a close friend, of a parent, of a spouse, of a child, leaves us crying out to an unfeeling universe in a plea for something to give meaning to our lives, and we search our souls to see if we have the strength to go on.

What gives meaning to the seemingly random and senseless tragedies in our lives is the realization that they are there for a purpose, even if at the time that purpose is a mystery wrapped in an enigma. It's really true that one door never closes without another one opening. As Ralph Waldo Emerson expressed it,

> *The compensations of calamity are made apparent to the understanding, after long periods of time. An illness, a cruel disappointment, a loss of wealth, a loss of friends, seems at the moment unpaid loss, and unpayable. But the sure years reveal the deep remedial force that underlies all facts.*

Or, as Boris Pasternak observed in *Dr. Zhivago*, "The virtue of people who have never fallen or stumbled is lifeless and isn't of much value. Life hasn't revealed its beauty to them."

I have a patient named Harry who last year lost his wife of thirty-four years, after a long bout with cancer. Harry had been devoted to Lillian, and was despondent. Week after week he would show up in my clinic, ostensibly to get his blood pressure checked, but in reality to look for some support. He would beseech me, "How can I go on? Nothing matters any more."

I tried in every way I could to console him, but nothing seemed to help. Finally, one day, I asked him, "Harry, suppose you had died first and Lillian had been alone. What would that have been like for her?" He was at first surprised by the question, but then said, "Why, she would have fallen to pieces. We were so close, it would have been too hard on her. And she didn't know anything about money, so she would have had to close our business. It's better this way."

"Well," I said, "then can you think of this as your gift to her? Hasn't the suffering *you've* gone through made it easier for *her*?" He said nothing as he left, but his brow was furrowed in thought.

For the next few weeks I didn't see him, but I heard that he was getting around more and had started going to meetings of his service club again. When he finally returned, he was almost his old self. "Doc," he said, "you know, I suddenly realized that this is just how I would have wanted it. We had a good life together, and I'm glad Lillian didn't have to go on without me. It *was* a lot easier on her this way." As he got up to leave, he fished something out of his pocket. "I want to give you this," he said. "She would have wanted you to have it. It meant a lot to her, those visits after she got cancer." He handed me a tattered old snapshot, a photo of the two of them at the Grand Canyon, a moment frozen in time when both were still young. I still have it on my office wall.

Another patient of mine, Chris, was never accepted by his parents because of his homosexuality. During his college years, his sexual identity became truly clear to him, and it was at that same time that his parents so completely disavowed his lifestyle that he began to visit them only those few times a year when it was unavoidable—usually just on birthdays and at Christmas. For more than a decade, he drifted helplessly away from his parents. Then, in his early thirties, he got AIDS.

"At first I thought that my parents would blame me," he told me, "and that they'd take an 'I-told-you-so' attitude. But along the way a miracle occurred, and that tragedy actually somehow brought us together again. I guess we all realized that it was our last chance. My mother would come to my apartment and cook for me, and my father helped me put some of my things into storage when I was too weak to do it. The communication and love and acceptance that opened up were incredible.

"Twice I nearly died of pneumocystis carinii pneumonia, and the second time, I'd actually surrendered to what seemed the inevitable, and I felt a deep peace and serenity," he continued. "Somehow, though, I pulled through. Even then, there were times when I was almost grateful for what had happened. The obvious miracle in my life was with my family, but I also realized that I was cherishing each day, that I was noticing the little things in life that I'd been too busy to appreciate before.

"And then a second miracle occurred," he recounted. "Ironically, within months of my acceptance that I wouldn't live to see the age of forty, the new triple antiviral therapy came out, and I've since almost completely rebounded. As you know, I'm back to my usual weight and almost all the energy I once had. Beyond the purely physical, though, I feel an inner strength that was never there before. I feel like I've been hammered on life's anvil into stronger steel. And what I have now I can give to others, and help them to be stronger too."

The poor but big-hearted Tevye in *A Fiddler on the Roof* suffers tragedies beyond what he thinks he can endure: grinding poverty, pogroms against his Jewish village, and, worst of all, a daughter who marries a gentile—an act that to him means losing her as a daughter forever. In despair, he flings his arms skyward and beseeches, "Why me, God?"

Yet finally, in his simple and moving faith, he turns to God again and says, "Thank You for these tragedies that have brought me closer to You," and picks up the reins of his horse cart and forges on.

If it weren't for life's storms that sometimes leave us feeling exhausted and hopeless, fearing that the next gargantuan wave will suck us under forever, never to see daylight again, life would be trite and superficial. It is those tempests that toss us about as the howling winds of life rage and blow, and we scramble for any scrap of flotsam that will keep us afloat, that test our courage and mettle, that allow us to exceed ourselves. If we can perceive the sea of life as our teacher, then we can see the beauty in the storms and realize that they are our guide. As Coleridge expressed it in *The Rime of the Ancient Mariner,*

> *The other was a softer voice,*
> *As soft as honey-dew:*
> *Quoth he, 'The man hath penance done,*
> *And penance more will do.'*
>
> *'But tell me, tell me! speak again,*
> *Thy soft response renewing—*
> *What makes that ship drive on so fast?*
> *What is the ocean doing?'*
>
> *'Still as a slave before his lord,*
> *The ocean hath no blast;*
> *His great bright eye most silently*
> *Up to the Moon is cast—*
>
> *'If he may know which way to go;*
> *For she guides him smooth or grim.*
> *See, brother, see! how graciously*
> *She looketh down on him.'*

CHAPTER NINETEEN

Does Anyone Actually Follow This Advice?

The program outlined in this book—regular exercise; a low-fat, low-cholesterol, high-fiber diet; a meaningful social support system; an avoidance of addictions; and a spiritual life that includes regular meditation—is so out of step with the average American's lifestyle that many will wonder if anyone can actually stick to such a program. This includes most physicians, many of whom are pessimistic about even getting their patients to stop smoking, let alone to eat right and exercise regularly.

And yet, in a remarkable achievement called the Opening Your Heart program, Dr. Dean Ornish, the author of *Dr. Dean Ornish's Program for Reversing Heart Disease,* asks his patients to do exactly that, and more. He asks his patients to do all of the above—plus daily yoga and daily guided visualization—and they *do* it.

The Ornish approach goes beyond simply promoting a social support system, and instead strives for true intimacy on the deepest levels. As Ornish describes it in his book,

> *At first I viewed our support groups simply as a way to motivate patients to stay on the other aspects of the program that I considered most important: the diet, exercise, stress management training, stopping smoking, and so on. Over time, I began to realize that the group support itself was one of the most powerful interventions, as it addressed what I am beginning to believe is a more fundamental cause of why we feel stressed, and, in turn, why we get illnesses like heart disease: the perception of isolation.*
>
> *In short, anything that promotes a sense of isolation leads to chronic stress and, often, to illnesses like heart disease. Conversely, anything that leads to real intimacy and feelings of connection can be healing in the real sense of the word: to make whole. The ability to be intimate has long been seen as a key to emotional health; I believe it is essential to the health of our hearts as well.*

The results? Starting with patients who are at high risk for heart attacks, most of whom have *already* had heart attacks, or at least angina, the Opening Your Heart program has cut the number of cardiac "events" in half compared to what would be expected with that group; it has decreased the number of fatal heart attacks to a tiny fraction of what it would otherwise be; and it has done so *not* by depriving the subjects in the program, but rather by dramatically *improving* the quality of their lives.

In my own spiritual community of Ananda, 350 people live in the mountains near Nevada City, California, and follow a lifestyle of meditation, vegetarianism, no smoking or alcohol, close community ties with a strong social support system, and at least minimal exercise by walking from place to place in the mountains. It was founded in 1968 as a spiritual community based on a nondenominational blend of Christian and Eastern religions, and includes meditation and yoga as the basis of the spiritual practices. The intention from the outset at Ananda was to found a spiritual community; although the health benefits of this lifestyle were always secondary, Ananda has inadvertently become a "laboratory" for the kind of program outlined in this book.

As visitors approach Ananda's guest facility, the Expanding Light, an aura of peace surrounds them from the moment they leave the car in the parking lot. The forested hills are dotted by lush gardens, and deer graze tranquilly in the surrounding meadows. From the Expanding Light building, uplifting music wafts gently over the lawn. Ananda's community members are a close and tight-knit group. With the exemplary health habits they practice, with an extraordinarily supportive social network, and with at least moderate exercise, almost all the adults look ten to fifteen years younger than their chronological ages, and almost all radiate positivity and idealism. The community takes to heart the saying "It takes a village to raise a child," and the many children of the community keep even the elders feeling young, with the kids knowing that all the adults they encounter know them and love them.

Ananda's Family Practice Clinic, founded in 1982 by my friend and mentor Dr. Peter Van Houten, is housed in a converted mobile home. Inside, in the simple but uplifting surroundings, longtime nurse practitioner Sue Loper-Powers talked to me about the health outcomes in this remarkable environment.

"We have an interesting point of view about the health of our community members, because most of the patients at our clinic don't come from the Ananda community, but rather from the surrounding hills. Part of the difference in health outcomes has to do with the different educational levels, because the Ananda people are a highly educated group, but I believe that a far greater part of the difference comes from the consciousness of our community people. We have only three smokers in the community that I know of, and we have some recovering alcoholics, but no one currently drinking.

"By contrast," she continued, "among our patients from outside the community, we see a remarkable amount of self-destructive activity, and some very unhappy people inhabiting some rapidly aging bodies. You're right that we didn't set out to promote health and longevity—Ananda has always been a fundamentally spiritual community—but one of the side effects of the lifestyle followed here is the extraordinary health of our community members.

"Nobody has ever kept statistics," she reflected, "but we believe that our heart attack rate is far below that of the outside world. The average age of the adults in the community is now around forty-five, yet most look a decade or two younger. Most of our people take antioxidants, and most of the women take calcium supplements, but otherwise the program is a simple one: daily meditation, vegetarian diet, exercise, an avoidance of addictions, and a very strong social support system. When people get sick, we have our HELP program: Healing Energy and Love Provided. If someone is sick, we can provide for someone to clean their house, drive them to the doctor, or pick up their medications. When a family has a baby, women from the community take turns bringing them a hot dinner. And, of course, the spiritual dimension of our community is integral to our health. If someone has a health issue, they can talk it over with one of the ministers and ask themselves, 'What's happening here?'

"So where's the trouble in paradise?" she replied to my question. "Well, despite our best efforts through the clinic, about a quarter of the people in the community are basically sedentary. And we certainly do have some lonely people, even here. Even with all the social supports, you can still be lonely if you don't make the effort."

The Ananda community welcomes visits from those who would like to see for themselves how the kind of program outlined in this book can be a reality. The Expanding Light guest facility offers seminars of from two days to more than a month, and a short tour can be arranged by simply showing up for Sunday services and then taking the traditional postservices guided tour.

The examples of both the Opening Your Heart program and the Ananda village make it clear that ordinary people can make extraordinary transformations in their lives; that many of the chronic "diseases of modern society" can be prevented or, when they do occur, even reversed; and that lifelong youthful living is within our grasp.

Perhaps equally important, though, is the common thread of these two examples—that a key factor in both has been the influence of a surrounding group of like-minded people to support transformation—or what at Ananda would be termed an "intentional community." Despite all the willpower we may bring to bear on a task, it is easy to become distracted if we are associating with people who don't share our vision and if we are surrounded by constant temptations. It is our communities that will make us whole.

The examples of the Opening Your Heart program and the Ananda community may seem inaccessible or too expensive for many, but even many small and isolated communities have low-cost or free support services for those seeking like-minded people. Most of America's small towns have Alcoholics Anonymous meetings and smoking-cessation and weight-loss support groups. And service groups and churches can be found everywhere.

We *can* make the changes we *must* make to transform our health and well-being. Those changes, far from being sacrifices or deprivations, actually result not just in a higher quality of life, but also in a true joyfulness in living. Our modern life has brought us many miracles of technology, but in many ways those changes have pulled us apart and made our lives more stressful. The high-technology medicine we now have has revolutionized our lives, but the real revolution may lie in simplifying our lives and once again living in the close communities we once knew.

CHAPTER TWENTY

Follow Your Dream

Of the many memorable patients I've seen, Emma is one of the most memorable. She was a seventy-three-year-old parochial school teacher who was sent by her principal to see me about back pain that she was experiencing "once in a while." We chatted briefly about the weather, but what really made her eyes light up was talking about her students. "They keep me young," she assured me.

Emma had the dowager's hump that is typical of a woman many years postmenopausal who has never taken estrogen. She agreed to an X ray, and when I put it on the view box, I was staggered. Emma had compression fractures of almost every vertebra, and many were subluxed, meaning they no longer rested properly on top of the next one.

My jaw dropped. My eyes kept going back and forth between Emma and her X ray. How was this woman even walking? Why wasn't she in excruciating pain?

The more I talked with her, though, the more I realized why: Emma had a purpose. Her children meant everything to her. The meaning they gave her overshadowed everything else in her life and allowed her to transcend the defects in her body that life had given her.

Emma finally agreed that maybe she would take some Tylenol from time to time. She then excused herself with a smile and a warm handshake, saying, "I need to get back to my kids." I had tears in my eyes as she left my exam room. I never saw her again.

Within all of us, no matter how well hidden, there dwells a dream—the fervent desire to make a contribution, to leave the world a better place than we found it, to know that it was not in vain that we trod upon this earth. As a physician, with the inestimable privilege of having an intimate window on the lives of so many people, I know that those who have lost their sense of meaning are so frail that they can be felled by a feather, while those who have a strong sense of purpose in their lives are indestructible and unstoppable—they just keep going.

Mother Teresa of Calcutta had medical problems that would have stopped a lesser person. She had severe congestive heart failure and her joints were crippled by arthritis. Yet that arthritis didn't stop her from grasping the hand of someone who desperately needed comforting and holding it close to her heart.

Although none of us may ever be a Mother Teresa, we all have some dream of helping others. For some of us, that means making our children the center of our lives; for others, it means helping out with our local youth group; for still others, it means simply planting a tree that will be there for generations to come. It is through such selfless acts that we transcend ourselves, that we go beyond the disappointments and disillusioning experiences that life has dealt us and recreate the idealism and exuberance that keep us young.

An ancient Zen koan says, "It is in losing yourself that you find yourself." Perhaps the Western version is from the Prayer of St. Francis: "It is in giving that we receive."

One of my inspirations, the great physician and spiritual leader Albert Schweitzer, said,

I don't know what your destiny will be, but one thing I do know: the only ones among you who will be truly happy will be those who have sought and found how to serve.

Richard Bach, the author of *Jonathan Livingston Seagull,* wrote, "Here's a test to find out if your mission on earth is finished: If you're alive, it isn't." Whatever wrong turns you may have taken in your life, whatever misfortunes may have befallen you, if you look deeply enough inside, you will still find that dream of making the world a better place burning brightly within.

Your chance to transcend yourself, to reconnect with that flame and to reach for the stars, lies in seeing your life as one of service, and of losing yourself in an ideal that is bigger than you are. If there is one last thought I would like to offer you in parting, it is to follow that dream, wherever it may lead you.

APPENDIX ONE

Summary of Recommendations

The following preventive health recommendations represent my own opinions. They lean strongly, however, on the recommendations of the American Academy of Family Practice and the Royal Canadian College of Family Practitioners.

Diet

- High-complex carbohydrate, high-fiber (fruits and vegetables), moderate protein, low-fat, low-cholesterol diet, eaten in frequent meals (four or five times a day) in small quantities.

Exercise

- At least one-half hour per day, five days a week, of vigorous aerobic exercise producing a heart rate near maximum, combined with weight-training exercise.

Health Supplements and Estrogen

- Vitamin C: 500 milligrams per day.

- Vitamin E: 600 international units (IU) per day.

- Selenium: 25 micrograms per day.

- Garlic extract: 1,500 milligrams per day.

- Flaxseed oil (for omega-3 fatty acids): 4,000 milligrams per day.

- Folate: 400 micrograms per day, especially for women of child-bearing age.

- Aspirin: one baby aspirin (81 milligrams) per day, for those over forty who have blood pressure in the normal range or controlled to normal, and no other risk factors for bleeding.

- Calcium: 500 to 1,000 milligrams per day, for women after onset of menopause.

- Estrogen: for almost all postmenopausal women, as prescribed by your physician.

Physical Examinations

- Physical examination yearly, including blood pressure and digital rectal exam (for prostate cancer in men and for colon cancer in both men and women), after age forty.

- *For women:* Pap and pelvic examination yearly, starting at age eighteen or when sexual activity begins, whichever comes first. Yearly manual breast examination by health care professional and monthly breast self-exam.

Lab Tests and Special Procedures

- Cholesterol screening in early adulthood, with appropriate follow-up if necessary. Cholesterol test every three years after age forty, for those in normal range.

- Fasting glucose test for diabetes, every three years after age forty-five, or earlier if symptoms of diabetes appear.

- TSH (thyroid-stimulating hormone) test for low thyroid, every three years after age forty, or earlier if symptoms of low thyroid appear.

- Three stool tests for fecal occult (hidden) blood every year after age forty.

- *For men:* PSA (prostate-specific antigen) test yearly after age fifty, or earlier if symptoms of prostate problems appear.

- *For women:* baseline mammogram in mid-thirties, followed by yearly mammogram after age forty, or earlier if risk factors are present.

Vaccinations

- *Influenza:* every year, starting at age four. It is very important for anyone at unusual risk for infectious diseases, such as those who have lost their spleen or who have emphysema or kidney failure. And it is highly recommended for anyone over sixty-five.

- *Pneumococcal pneumonia:* once, for anyone over fifty. Also for all younger people who are at unusual risk for infectious diseases, such as those mentioned above. (Do not confuse this vaccine for adults with a different pneumococcal vaccine recently developed for children; the latter is aimed at preventing meningitis, and it will also reduce ear infections.)

- *Tetanus:* every ten years.

Meditation

- Meditation for at least fifteen minutes per day, preferably preceded by a warm-up with yoga or other relaxation exercises.

Spiritual Life

- Regular devotional activities, per your own beliefs.

℘ ℘ ℘

A last word from a veteran emergency physician: Please make the time to donate blood regularly, and don't forget to sign your organ donor card. Although you will probably never meet them, there are people out there whose lives depend on your generosity.

APPENDIX TWO

Recommended Reading &

Stay Young, Start Now is a medical book written by a generalist. Much of what is discussed in it will lead to an interest to further pursue the subject. What follows are recommendations of books written by recognized authorities, and that generally follow the medical philosophy outlined in *Stay Young, Start Now*.

Alcohol Dependence

Al J. Mooney, M.D., Arlene Eisenberg & Howard Eisenberg, *The Recovery Book*, Workman Publishing, 1992

Written by a physician with multiple family members who have alcohol issues. Complete and accurate—this book could well become a classic in its field.

Breasts

Yashar Hirshaut, M.D., F.A.C.P., Peter I. Pressman, M.D., F.A.C.S., *Breast Cancer The Complete Guide*, Bantam, 1996

Written by a surgeon and an internist, this book does an excellent job of addressing all of the modalities of treating breast cancer: surgery, radiation therapy, chemotherapy, and hormonal therapy, as well as discussing prevention strategies.

Diabetes

Diabetes is a subject barely touched on in *Stay Young, Start Now*, as it is a book-length subject in itself. The following are excellent books on the subject for the nonmedical general public:

American Diabetes Association Complete Guide to Diabetes, The authoritative Resource from the Diabetes Experts, *American Diabetes Association,* 1997

This book truly is complete and authoritative, and should be the first place to look for support with diabetes.

David S. Schade, M.D., Editor in Chief, Patrick J. Boyle, M.D., and others. 101 Tips for Staying Healthy with Diabetes (& Avoiding Complications), *American Diabetes Association,* 1996

Written and produced by the University of New Mexico Diabetes Care Team, this is an excellent companion to the ADA "Complete Guide."

Judith Wylie-Rosett, EdD, R.D., Charles Swencionis, Ph.D., and others, The Complete Weight Loss Workbook Proven Techniques for Controlling Weight-Related Health Problems, *American Diabetes Association,* 1997

Maintaining ideal weight is especially crucial to diabetics, but is a challenge because of the risk of hypoglycemia (low blood sugar). This book provides clear and accurate information.

Diet

Dean Ornish, M.D., *Eat More, Weigh Less* Harper Collins, 1993

Here Dr. Ornish explains his low-fat heart health diet that has the happy effect of producing weight loss in most of those who follow the diet carefully.

Harvey and Marilyn Diamond, *Fit for Life,* Warner Books, 1985

Harvey and Marilyn Diamond, *Fit for Life II: Living Health, The Complete Health Program,* Warner Books, 1987

A classic best-seller, Fit for Life *and its sequel are especially strong as motivators. Their advice about avoiding mixing certain foods has little scientific basis—but, it won't hurt, either.*

Exercise

Robert Arnot, M.D., *Guide to Turning Back the Clock*, Little, Brown and Company, 1995

An excellent motivator that also makes the case for both cardiovascular fitness and weight training. Primarily aimed at men.

Bob Greene and Oprah Winfrey, *Make the Connection: Ten Steps to a Better Body and a Better Life*, Hyperion, 1996

Another excellent motivator with a solid conditioning program. Written by the well-known daytime TV host, this book may be especially appreciated by women.

Family Practice

Heirs of General Practice by John McPhee, Noonday Press, 1991

The classic on the "specialty" of family practice and the last of the truly generalist family physicians. The family practitioners profiled in McPhee's book do not also practice emergency medicine, as the author of Stay Young, Start Now and many other family practitioners do.

Heart Disease

Dr. Dean Ornish, M.D., *Dr. Dean Ornish's Program for Reversing Heart Disease*, Ivy Books, 1996

A breakthrough book by one of the most influential physicians of our time, this book is required reading for anyone with heart disease.

Michael E. DeBakey, M.D. & Antonio M. Gotto, Jr., M.D., *The New Living Heart*, Adams Media Corporation, 1997

The New Living Heart *is oriented primarily toward surgical treatments of heart disease. Written by one of the great pioneers in the field.*

Hysterectomy

Winnifred B. Cutler, Ph.D., *Hysterectomy: Before and After*, HarperPerennial, 1990

The best book on weighing the pros and cons of hysterectomy, this book advocates avoiding the procedure where possible.

Recommended Reading

Meditation

John Novak, *How to Meditate,* Crystal Clarity Press, 1992

Menopause

Winnifred B. Cutler, Ph.D. & Celso-Ramón García, M.D., *Menopause—A Guide for Women & Those Who Love Them,* Norton & Company, 1993

Written by the two ideal authorities on the subject—a renowned reproductive endocrinologist and a research obstetrician and gynecologist.

Geoffrey Redmond, M.D., *The Good News About Women's Hormones,* Warner Books, 1995

A somewhat technical book written by an endocrinologist.

Susan Rako, M.D. *The Hormone of Desire-The Truth About Sexuality, Menopause and Testosterone,* Harmony Books, 1996

Presents extremely interesting new information about the central importance of testosterone to the female libido.

Mary Jane Minkin, M.D. *What Every Woman Needs to Know About Menopause: The Years Before, During and After,* Yale University Press, 1996

Written by a gynecologist with twenty years' experience, this book covers both the physiologic and psychological aspects of menopause.

Penny Wise Budoff, M.D. *No More Hot Flashes...And Even More Good News,* Warner Books, 1998

Written by a specialist in women's health. Excellent coverage of the new "designer hormone" Evista.

Osteoporosis

Susan E. Brown, Ph.D., *Better Bones,* Better Body Kent Publishing, 1996

A holistic approach to bone health written by a medical anthropologist and nutritionist.

Alan R. Gaby, M.D. *Preventing and Reversing Osteoporosis,* Prima Health, 1994

Another holistic approach to bone health with a heavy emphasis on nutrition. Contains perhaps too enthusiastic a recommendation of DHEA.

Prostate

Sheldon Marks, M.D., *Prostate & Cancer—A Family Guide to Diagnosis, Treatment & Survival,* Fisher Books, 1995

A superb treatment of prostate cancer and benign prostatic hypertrophy with an excellent question and answer section.

Smoking Cessation

Terry A. Rustin, M.D., *Quit & Stay Quit. A personal Program to Stop Smoking* Hazelden, 1994

Written by a physician who conducts seminars and workshops on nicotine dependence, and who is the Texas Chair of the American Society of Addiction Medicine. A clear, systematic approach to stopping smoking and staying stopped.

Social Support System

Dr. Dean Ornish, M.D., *Love & Survival,* HarperPerennial, 1999

Dr. Ornish to the rescue again. This landmark book documents the many scientific studies showing a profound link between our social support systems and mortality rates.

Women's Health

Christiane Northrup, M.D., *Women's Bodies, Women's Wisdom,* Bantam Books, 1994

A classic, in-depth book on women's health that addresses not just the physical but the spiritual.

Nancy Snyderman, M.D., *Dr. Nancy Snyderman's Guide to Good Health for Women Over Forty,* Harcourt Brace & Company, 1996

Medically accurate, although a little on the dry side, this book addresses a broad range of issues affecting women over forty.

The Internet and Health

The Internet has been in some ways a breakthrough for health care, allowing patients to communicate with others with the same health issues via support groups, and allowing physicians rapid access to medical literature searches and the ability to consult with other physicians about difficult cases. In some ways, how-

Recommended Reading

ever, the internet has been a curse, as it has allowed anonymous people to log-on and offer dubious medical advice.

A good place to start would be Dr. Dean Edell's very extensive site with information on a very wide range of medical issues. The web site address is: *http://www.dredell.com*. Then click on health central. You can also go directly to this web site where you will find Dr. Edell: http://www.healthcentral.com

Dr. Koop

http://www.drkoop.com/wellness and to read his biography go to: *http://www.collphyphil.org/koopbio.htm*

Breast Cancer

The Mayo Clinic web site for breast cancer.

http://www.mayohealth.org/mayo/9609/htm/breast_c.htm

The American Cancer Society web site for breast cancer.

http://www2.cancer.org/bcn

Cancer

The American Cancer Society web site. This is the home page

http://www.cancer.org

Diabetes

The American Diabetes Association

http://www.diabetes.org

Another interesting web site with a lot of information

http://www.diabetes.com

Heart Disease

The American Heart Association home page

http://www.americanheart.org

The American Heart Association for women

http://www.women.americanheart.org

Menopause

The North American Menopause Society

http://www.menopause.org

Osteoporosis

The Osteoporosis Center. It is located in Modesto, California.

http://www.sonnet.com/usr/imaging

The National Osteoporosis Foundation

http://www.nof.org

Prostate

The American Prostate Society

http://www.ameripros.org

This site has information on prostate cancer, prostate enlargement and other health problems with the prostate.

Smoking Cessation

Foundation for Innovations in Nicotine Dependence

http://www.findhelp.com

This is the web site of about.com where you can obtain a lot of information on smoking cessation.

http://www.quitsmoking.about.com

The American Lung Association

http://www.lungusa.org

At the bottom of the page, on the right hand site corner, there is a window that says "Search the Entire Site." Type "smoke cessation" and then click "search."

INDEX

A
Abdominal aorta, Plate 1
Acetaminophen, 178
Active listening, 226
Addictions, 7, 51. *See also*
 Alcohol use; Drug use;
 Smoking
 meditation and, 248
Adoption, 132–134
Advil. *See* Ibuprofen
Aerobics classes, 200
AIDS, 18, 254–255
 sexuality and, 119
Alcoholics Anonymous, 204,
 213–215, 262
 founders of, 219
 higher power in, 244
Alcohol use, 203–204
 as addiction, 212–220
 fertility issues and, 130
 gastric ulcers and, 179
 health affects of, 214–215
 heart attacks and, 217–219
 osteoporosis and, 145
 pregnancy and, 126
 ReVia, 218
 sexual function (male) and,
 101
 weight loss and, 201
Alendronate, 140
Alfalfa sprouts, 145
Alpha-1 blockers, 105–106
Alprostadil, 108
Alternative medical providers,
 230
Alzheimer's disease, 37
 alcohol use and, 217
 aspirin and, 178
 DHEA and, 185
 estrogen replacement and,
 139
 social isolation and, 71–72
Ambivalence, 68–69
American Cancer Society,
 167–168
*American Diabetes Association
 Complete Guide to
 Diabetes* (Kahn), 170

Amniocentesis, 124
Amphetamines and weight loss,
 194
Amyotrophic lateral sclerosis
 (Lou Gehrig's disease), 55
Ananda, 259–262
 Family Practice Clinic, 260
 HELP program, 261
Anesthesia, 239, 241
Angina, 19, 25, Plate 3
 coronary bypass surgery,
 236
Angioplasty, 24, 236
 emergency procedure, 163
 Mayo Clinic study, 55
 risk of, 237
Animal products, 192–193
Ankylosing spondylitis, 60
Anorexia, 189, 195, 205
Antabuse, 218
Antibiotics, 17
Antidepressants, 59
 sexual function (male) and,
 104
Antihistamines, 104
Antioxidants, 175–177
 in animal products, 192
Antipsychotics, 59
Aorta, 19, Plate 3
 abdominal aorta, Plate 1
 thoracic aorta, Plate 1
Aortic aneurysms, 28
Apomorphine, 100
Armstrong, Lance, 55, 161
Arthritis, 203
 omega-3 fatty acids and, 182
Ascites, 214
Aspirin
 baby aspirin, 180
 gastric ulcers and, 179
 hemorrhagic stroke and, 183
Asthma, 86
Atelectasis, 241
Athena Institute, 118
Atherosclerosis, 29
 free radicals and, 175
 garlic and, 184
 Viagra and, 96

Atrial fibrillation, 22–23, Plate 3
 clots and, 25
Atrial flutter, 23, Plate 3
Atrioventricular node, 19,
 Plate 2, Plate 3
Autonomic nervous system,
 100–101
Autosomal chromosomes,
 127–128

B
Back pain, 238–239
 surgeries for, 238, 240
Bacteria, garlic and, 184
Bacterial prostatitis, 159
Barrier contraception, 129
Basal-cell carcinomas, 170
Beatty, Warren, 90
Bedside manner, 226
Beef, 46
Benign prostatic hyperplasia
 (BPH), 159–160
 Cardura for, 105
Bennett, William, 207
Benzodiazepines
 sexual function (female) and,
 117
 sexual function (male) and,
 104
Beta-blockers, 104
Beta-carotene, 175
Bile salts, 44
Birth. *See* Childbirth
Bladder
 in female, Plate 5
 in male, Plate 6
Blood clots, 25
 estrogen and, 148–149
 Evista and, 143
 obesity and, 191
Blood donations, 20–21, 269
Bloodletting, 20–21
Blood pressure. *See also* High
 blood pressure
 checking on, 165–166
 weight and, 190
Blood thinners, 20–21, 163
 vitamin E and, 176

277

Body Mass Index (BMI), 30–31
  life expectancy and, 23
Bone health. *See* Osteoporosis
Brain. *See also* Strokes
  blood supply of, Plate 4
Breast cancer, 137–138
  cure rates for, 138
  estrogen and, 142, 148–149
  Evista and, 143
  exercise and, 38
  fiber and, 44, 45
  mortality rate, 155
  obesity and, 191
  tamoxifen and, 138, 143
  Xenical and, 195
Breast Cancer: The Complete Guide (Hirshaut & Pressman), 138
Brindley, Giles, 109
Bulimia, 189, 195, 205
Bupropion, 209
Bypass surgery. *See* Coronary bypass surgery

C
Calan, 106
Calcitonin, 140
Calcium channel blockers, 106
Calcium supplements, 144–145, 147–148
Calories, 46
Cancer, 17, 32–33. *See also* Metastasis; specific types
  alcohol use and, 214
  animal products and, 192
  estrogen and, 148–149
  exercise and, 38
  free radicals and, 175
  garlic and, 184
  hysterectomies and, 150
  melatonin and, 186
  unmarried persons with, 72
Caput medusae, 214
Car accidents, 18
  alcohol use and, 215
Cardiovascular exercise, 39
Cardiovascular system, Plate 1
Cardura
  for benign prostatic hyperplasia (BPH), 159–160
  congestive heart failure and, 106
  sexual function (male) and, 105

Carnegie Mellon University study, 73
Carotid arteries, Plate 3, Plate 4
Car shades, 172
Catapress, 104
Cats, 87
Caverject, 96, 108–109
Cereals, folate in, 181
Cervical cancer, 135–136
  mortality rate, 155
  sexual activity and, 136
Cervical caps, 129
  cervical cancer, prevention of, 136
Cervix. *See also* Cervical cancer
  hysterectomies and, 150, 151–152
  os, 152
  sensitivity of, 152–153
Cesarean sections, 127, 238
Chemotherapy, 138
Chicken, 46
Childbirth, 121–122. *See also* Fertility issues
  mortality and, 18
  thirty-five, risks after, 126–128
Children, 121–134
  adoption, 132–134
  death of, 131–132
  touch and, 87
Chiropractors, 86
  back pain and, 238
Chlamydia, 125
Cholesterol
  drugs for lowering, 26–27
  exercise and, 37
  fiber and, 44–45
  garlic and, 184
  heart attacks and, 19, 180–181
  human growth hormone and, 187
  meditation and, 248
  melatonin and, 186
  omega-3 fatty acids and, 182
  screening, 166
  sexual function (male) and, 93, 94
  Slo-Niacin for, 27
  testosterone replacement and, 115
Chromosomes
  autosomal chromosomes, 127–128

  sex chromosomes, 116, 128
Chronic fatigue syndrome, 185
Chronological age, 9
Cigarettes. *See* Smoking
Cigars, 207–208
Circle of Willis, 28, Plate 4
Cirrhosis of the liver, 214
Clitoris, 116
Clot-busting drugs, 24, 25
Cocaine, 117
Codependency, 216
Coffee, osteoporosis and, 145
Colonoscopy, 167–168
Colorectal cancer
  aspirin and, 178–181
  estrogen replacement and, 141
  fiber and, 32, 44, 45
  obesity and, 191
  rectal exams and, 137
  screening for, 166–168
  spiritual life and, 243
Communication
  erectile dysfunction and, 98–99
  health and, 69–70
  Holocaust survivors and, 80–82
  openness in, 8
Commuting, exercise and, 42
Condoms, 128
  cervical cancer, prevention of, 136
Congestive heart failure, 17
  alcohol use and, 214
  arrhythmias and, 23–24
  Cardura and, 106
  exercise and, 37
Contraception, 129. *See also* specific types
Cooper, Kenneth, 175–176
Coronary arteries, 19, Plate 3
  electrical system of heart, 22
  exercise and, 37
  hematocrit and, 20–21
Coronary bypass surgery, 25, 236–237
  frequency of, 238–239
Corpus callosum, 64
Coumadin
  aspirin and, 180
  omega-3 fatty acids and, 183
  vitamin E and, 176
Couric, Katie, 166–167
Cousins, Norman, 231

Index

Culturally related illnesses, 61
Cutler, Winnifred, 154–155
Cycling progesterone/estrogen, 146

D
Dartmouth Medical School study, 244–245
Death
 of child, 131–132
 dealing with, 252
 risks for, 15–33
Delirium tremens, 215
Demerol, 204
Depression
 alcoholism and, 215
 exercise and, 38–39
 heart attacks and, 55
 hysterectomies and, 154
 Internet use and, 73
 meditation and, 248
 melatonin and, 186
 menopause and, 13
 resistance to illness and, 69
 sexual function (male) and, 103
 smoking and, 67, 206
 touch and, 86
Desyrel, 104–105
 sexual function (male) and, 104–105
DHEA (dehydroepiandrosterone), 184–185
DHT, 160
Diabetes
 estrogen replacement and, 141
 exercise and, 38
 fiber and, 44
 gestational diabetes, 126
 juvenile-onset, 203
 low-fat diet and, 46
 screening for, 169–170
 sexual function (male) and, 94
 sexual relations and, 102
 vascular disease and, 29
 weight and, 190
Diaphragms, 129
 cervical cancer, prevention of, 136
Diet. *See also* High-fat diet
 benefits of, 51
 healthful diet, 44–53

 protein sources in, 46–47
 recommendations for, 266
 sexual function (female) and, 116–117
 sexual function (male) and, 94
 starting healthful diet, 48
 vegetarian diet, 192–193
Digoxin, 104
Dilantin, 104
Disk surgeries, 240
Disulfiram, 218
Diverticulitis, 45
Diverticulosis, fiber and, 45
Dogs, 87
Double-blind studies, 173–174, 176–177
Dowager's hump, 141
Down's syndrome, 127
Doxazosin. *See* Cardura
Dr. Dean Ornish's Program for Reversing Heart Disease (Ornish), 257–258
Drug use, 204. *See also* Heroin; Medications
 sexual function (female) and, 117
Duodenal ulcers, 179
Dupuytren's contractures, 215
Dyazide, 104

E
Ectopic pregnancies, 125
Electrocardiograms, 164
Embolic stroke, 25
Emergency physicians, 227
Emotional Quotient, 162–163
Empty-nesters, 122
Endometrial biopsies, 151, 152
Endometrial cancer, 135–136
 estrogen replacement and, 142
Endometriosis, 125
 hysterectomies and, 150
Endorphins
 exercise and, 39
 sexual relations and, 93
 uterus producing, 154
Epidural anesthesia, 239, 241
Epilepsy, 64
Erecaid, 110
Erections. *See* Sexual function (male)
Esophageal cancer, 214

Essential hypertension, 126
Estrace, 147
Estradiol, 147
Estrogen, 116–117, 139–149
 breast cancer and, 142, 148–149
 contraindications to, 148–149
 cycling with progesterone, 146–147
 declining treatment with, 144–145
 exercise and, 38
 heart attack risk and, 140–141
 hysterectomies and, 154
 menopause and, 115
 recommendations for, 267
 side effects of, 147
Evista, 143
Exercise
 angina and, 19
 benefits of, 37–43, 51
 heart attacks and, 24
 hunger and, 194
 levels of, 190
 osteoporosis and, 149
 recommendations for, 266
 regularity of, 43
 self-assessment, 40–41
 sexual function (female) and, 116–117
 sexual function (male) and, 94
 smoking and, 211
 starting program of, 48
 surgery and, 241
 weight loss and, 201
Expanding Light, Ananda, 259, 261

F
Fallopian tubes, 124–125
 hysterectomies and, 150
Family nurse practitioners (FNPs), 229
Family practitioners, 227–228
Fasting glucose test, 169
Fecal occult blood tests, 168
Feet
 circulation in, 28–29
 as vulnerable point, Plate 1
Femur, osteoporotic/healthy, Plate 7
Fenfluramine, 194
Fertility issues, 123–124, 129

279

advice on, 129–131
obesity and, 191
Fiber, 22, 44–45
   colon cancer and, 32, 44, 45, 167
   diabetes and, 44
   diverticulosis and, 45
Fibroids, 150
Finasteride, 160
Fish, 46–47
Fish oils. *See* Omega-3 fatty acids
Fixx, Jimmy, 17
Flatus, 195
Flaxseed oil, 181–182
Flu vaccinations, 268
Folate
   homocysteine levels and, 180
   pregnancy and, 181
   supplements, 124, 128
Food. *See also* Diet; High-fat diet
   emotional connection to, 195, 198
Food and Drug Administration (FDA)
   on folate, 181
   weight loss drugs, 194
Fosamax, 140
Framingham Study, 26
Free radicals, 175–176
   exercise and, 43
   garlic and, 184
Freud, Sigmund, 12
   talking cure, 62
Fruits, 22
Fusions, 238, 240

G
Galen, 55, 58, 183
Gallbladder
   estrogen and, 148–149
   obesity and gallstones, 191
Gambling, 205
Garlic supplements, 183–184
Gastric ulcers, 179
   alcohol use and, 214
General anesthesia, 239, 241
Geritol, 177
Gestational diabetes, 126
Gilda's Club, 135
Glaser, Jay, 185
Goals, setting, 6–7
Gonorrhea, 125
Grinkov, Sergei, 17

H
Haldol, 65
Hamilton, Scott, 161
Happiness, 12
Harvard School of Public Health study, 32
Hawking, Stephen, 54–55
Health care providers, 221–233
Health clubs, 42
Health maintenance organizations (HMOs), 221
Heart. *See also* Congestive heart failure; Coronary bypass surgery
   blood flow through, Plate 2
   electrical conduction system, blood supply to, Plate 3
   pumping action of, Plate 2
   as vulnerable site, Plate 1
Heart attacks, 1–4, 12, 17
   alcohol use and, 217–219
   in Ananda community, 260
   arrhythmias and, 23–24
   aspirin and, 178–181
   causes of, 18–19
   damage from, 24
   depression and, 55
   estrogen and, 117
   exercise and, 37
   fish oils and, 181–183
   garlic and, 184
   homocysteine and, 180–181
   iron and, 21
   meditation and, 248
   men and, 161–164
   menopause and, 140–141, 152
   Pickwickian syndrome, 191
   self-assessment of risks, 56–58
   symptoms of, 163–164
   thinning of blood and, 20–21
   thyroid and, 169
   water and, 20
   weight and, 190–191
   in women, 152–153
Hefner, Hugh, 90
Heirs of General Practice (McPhee), 228
Hematocrit, 20–21
Hemochromatosis, 21
Hemorrhagic stroke, 25, 28
   aspirin and, 179
   omega-3 fatty acids and, 183
Hepburn, Audrey, 166

Heroin
   sexual function (female) and, 117
   smoking and, 208
High blood pressure
   congestive heart failure and, 24
   essential hypertension, 126
   medications and sexual function, 105
   Meridia and, 195
   pregnancy and, 126–127
   as risk factor, 29
   sexual function (male) and, 94
   symptoms of, 166
   vascular disease and, 29
High-density lipoprotein (HDL), 115
High-fat diet
   breast cancer and, 138
   cancer and, 32, 138
   health consequences of, 50
   obesity and, 193–194
   prostate cancer and, 158
   vascular disease and, 29
Hip fracture, Plate 7
Hippocrates, 84
Hirshaut, Yashar, 138
Holocaust survivors, 80–82
Homocysteine, 180–181
Homosexuality, 254
Honduras, prostate cancer in, 158
Hormonal system, 102–103
Hospitals, social isolation and, 72–75
Hot flashes, 139
   Evista and, 143
How to Meditate (Novak), 248
Human growth hormone, 187–188
Human papilloma virus, 136
Hunger, exercise and, 194
Hunzas of Pakistan, 193
Hydrochlorothiazide, 104
Hydrocodone, 117
Hypertension. *See* High blood pressure
Hypothyroidism, 169
Hysterectomies, 92, 150–155
   cycling estrogen and progesterone after, 146–147
   depression and, 154
   estrogen replacement and, 154
   need for, 238

Index

Hysterectomy: Before and After (Cutler), 154–155
Hytrin, 159–160
  sexual function (male) and, 106

I

Ibuprofen, 178
  gastric ulcers and, 179
Immune system
  meditation and, 248
  melatonin and, 186
  omega-3 fatty acids and, 182
  vitamin C and, 176
Impotence. See Sexual function (male)
Inderal, 104
Infant mortality, 18
Inferior vena cava, 19, Plate 3
Infertility. See Fertility issues
Influenza vaccinations, 268
Insomnia
  estrogen replacement and, 141
  meditation and, 248
  melatonin and, 186
  Zyban and, 209
Internet
  as addiction, 205
  depression and, 73
Intestines, Plate 1
Intimacy, 69
Inuit of Greenland, 182, 183
Iron
  heart attacks and, 21
  supplements, 177
Irritable bowel syndrome, 62–63

J

Japan
  heart attack rate in, 182
  prostate cancer in, 158
Jet lag, 186
Jewish General Hospital, Montreal, 77, 80–82, 226
Johns Hopkins School of Public Health study, 55
Journal of the Royal Society of Medicine, 243
Junk foods, 46, 190

K

Kahn, Richard, 170
Kegel exercises, 118

Kidneys
  arteries, Plate 1
  vascular disease and, 29
Kidney stones, 21
  vitamin C and, 176
Kinsey studies, 91
Klinefelter's syndrome, 128

L

Laboratory tests, recommendations for, 268
Lamb, 46
Laminectomies, 238, 240
Lanoxin, 104
Lemieux, Mario, 55
Libido
  age and, 91
  DHEA and, 184
  hysterectomies and, 151
  menopause and, 116
Librium
  sexual function (female) and, 117
  sexual function (male) and, 104
Life expectancy
  Body Mass Index (BMI) and, 30–31
  evaluating you, 22–23
  in 1900, 18
Lifestyle. See also Sedentary lifestyle
  factors in healthy lifestyle, 36
  risks and, 16
  sexual function (female) and, 116–117
  sun exposure and, 171–172
The Light of Consciousness (Mann), 249
Linseed oil, 181–182
Liver
  alcohol use and, 214
  cirrhosis of, 214
  colon cancer and, 167
  estrogen and disease, 148–149
  ReVia and, 218
Loper-Powers, Sue, 260
Lortab, 117
Love, Medicine and Miracles (Siegel), 54
Lumpectomy, 138
Lung cancer, 152
Lungs, 19, Plate 1
Lycopene, 158

M

McGill School of Medicine, 226–227
  Osler and, 245
McPhee, John, 228
Macular degeneration, 206
Magnesium, 145
Mammary arteries, 25
Mammograms, 137
  radiation exposure from, 138
Manganese, 145
Mann, Richard D., 249
Marks, Sheldon, 161
Massage therapists, 86
Mastectomy, 138
Masters and Johnson studies, 91
Maya, 251
Mayo Clinic angioplasty study, 55
Mead Johnson, 147
Medicaid, 224
Medical schools, 222–226
Medicare, 224
Medications. See also specific types
  for benign prostatic hyperplasia (BPH), 159–160
  fertility drugs, 129
  sexual function (male) and, 104–110
  for weight loss, 194–195
Meditation
  benefits of, 51, 246–250
  fertility and, 131
  melatonin and, 187
  recommendations for, 269
  surgery and, 241
Melanoma, 170
  illustration, Plate 8
Melatonin, 186–187
Memory. See also Alzheimer's disease
  alcohol use and, 215
  DHEA and, 184
  exercise and, 37
Menopause, 112–113, 139–149
  heart attacks and, 140–141, 152
  medical school classes on, 223
Mental illness, 59
Meperidine, 204
Meridia, 195
Mesenteric infarction, 28
Mesenteric ischemia, Plate 1

Mesenteric vascular insufficiency, 28
Metastasis, 136
  breast cancer and, 137–138
  of colon cancer, 167
Mexican-Americans, 74
Miacalcin, 140
Migraine headaches, 86
Mind/body connection, 53, 55, 58
  culturally related illnesses, 61–62
  in medical schools, 222–223
Mind/mind connection, 53
Monahan, Jay, 166
Montessori, Maria, 12
Mood swings, 139
Motrin. *See* Ibuprofen
Multiple births, 127
Multiple personality disorder (MPD), 65–67
Multiple sclerosis, 182
Multivitamins, 177
Murder, 18
  meditation and, 248
Muscles, DHEA and, 184
Muse, 108

N
Naltrexone, 218
The Natural History of Alcoholism (Vaillant), 244
Navajo Indians, 61–62
  traditional medicine of, 231–232
Nervous system
  meditation and, 248
  sexual function (male) and, 100–102
New England Journal of Medicine, 238
New Passages (Sheehy), 9, 114
Niacin, 27
Nicotine addiction. *See* Smoking
Nicotine patches/chewing gum, 210
Nicotinic acid, 27
Nitroglycerin, Viagra and, 97
Novak, John, 248

O
Oatmeal, cholesterol and, 44–45
Obesity, 47, 189–202
  alcohol use and, 215
  diabetes and, 170
  emotional component and, 195
  fertility issues and, 130
  genetics and, 192
  support groups, 195, 198
  vascular disease and, 29
Obstetrician-gynecologists, 228–229
Omega-3 fatty acids, 47, 181–183
  hemorrhagic stroke and, 183
Opening Your Heart program, 257–258, 261–262
Ophthalmic artery, Plate 4
Oral sex, 99
  preference for, 107
Organ donor cards, 269
Orgasm
  antidepressants and, 104–1057
  exercise and, 38
  hysterectomies and, 151
  in postmenopausal women, 116, 117
  Viagra and, 96
Orlistat, 195
Ornish, Dean, 16, 237, 257–258
Orthopedists, 86
Osler, William, 32, 244, 245–246
Os of cervix, 152
Osteoporosis, 141
  diagram of osteoporotic bones, Plate 7
  exercise and, 38, 149
  Fosamax for, 140
  Miacalcin for, 140
  smoking and, 145, 149, 206
  vitamin supplements and, 145
  weight training and, 39
Ova, 124
Ovarian cancer, 135–136
  hysterectomies and, 150, 151
  obesity and, 191
Ovaries, 137, Plate 5
  hysterectomies and, 150
Overweight. *See* Obesity
Ovulation, 130
Oxycodone, 117

P
Papaverine, 109
Pap exams, 135, 136–137

Parasympathetic nervous system, 100–101
  meditation and, 248
Parkinson's disease, 141
Passive smoke, 206
Pasteur, Louis, 183, 245
Pauling, Linus, 176
Paxil, 104
Pediatricians, 227
Pelvic exams, 135–137
Pelvic inflammatory disease (PID), 124–125
Penile artery, 94, Plate 6
Penile implants, 110
Penis, Plate 6. *See also* Priapism; Sexual function (male)
Percocet, 117
Peripheral vascular disease, 28–29
Personal trainers, 42
Phentolamine, 100, 109–110
Pheromones, 118
Physical examinations, 267
Physical therapists, 43
Physician assistants (PAs), 229
Physician-patient relationships, 223
Physicians' Health Study, 179
Phytoestrogens, 145
Pickwickian syndrome, 191
Pineal gland, 186
Placebo effect, 77, 174
Placebos, 174
  Zyban and, 209
Pneumonia, 17–18
  as postoperative complication, 241
  vaccinations for, 268–269
Polycythemia vera, 20–21
Pondimin, 194
Pork, 46
Preeclampsia, 126–127
Pregnancy. *See also* Childbirth; Fertility issues
  ectopic pregnancies, 125
  in forties, 123–124
  preeclampsia, 126–127
  smoking and, 206
  social support and, 72
Premarin. *See* Estrogen
Premature infants, 83–84
  older mothers and, 127
Premenstrual syndrome (PMS), 150

Index

Pressman, Peter, 138
Priapism, 97
  Desyrel and, 105
Progesterone
  breast cancer and, 142
  cycling with estrogen, 146–147
  endometrial cancer and, 142
  side effects of, 147
Prolixin, 65
Prometrium, 147
Proscar, 160
Prospective studies, 174
Prostate and Cancer: A Family Guide to Diagnosis, Treatment, and Survival (Marks), 161
Prostate cancer
  obesity and, 191
  prevention of, 158
  screening for, 157–158
  selenium and, 177
  sexual relations and, 93
  treatment of, 160
Prostate gland, 157–161, 158
  symptoms of problem, 158
Prostate-specific antigen (PSA), 159
Protein, 144–145
Provera. *See* Progesterone
Prozac, 194–195
  sexual function (male) and, 104
Psychiatric illness. *See also* Depression
  Mexican-Americans and, 74
  multiple personality disorder (MPD), 65–67
  schizophrenia, 65
Psychiatrists, 59
Pubococcygeal muscle, 118
Pulmonary arteries/veins, 19
Pulmonary emboli, 28
P-waves, Plate 2

Q
Quinn, Janet, 87

R
Radiation therapy, 102
  for breast cancer, 138
  for prostate cancer, 160
Radner, Gilda, 135
Raloxifene, 143

Randomized studies, 176
Raynaud's disease, 106
Rectal cancer. *See* Colorectal cancer
Rectal exams, 137
  for colon cancer, 167
  for prostate problems, 158–159
Rectum. *See also* Colorectal cancer
  in female, Plate 5
  in male, Plate 6
Red meats, 46
Redux, 194
Relationships
  communication and, 76–77
  goals for, 7
Renal artery vascular disease, 29
Repeatable studies, 178
Research, 175–178
Resistance to illness, 69
ReVia, 218
Risks, 15–33
Running, 39, 42

S
Salmon, 47
Salt, osteoporosis and, 145
Saphenous vein, 25
Schulz, Charles, 12, 166
Schweitzer, Albert, 183, 265
Second adulthood, 114
Sedentary lifestyle
  breast cancer and, 138
  health consequences of, 50
  obesity and, 193–194
  vascular disease and, 29
Selenium
  as antioxidant, 175, 176–177
  prostate cancer and, 158
Self-transformation, 9, 12
SERMS (selective estrogen receptor modulators), 143
Serotonin-reuptake inhibitors, 104
Serum, 20–21
Sex chromosomes, 116, 128
Sexual abuse
  eating disorders and, 195
  irritable bowel syndrome and, 62–63
  multiple personality disorder (MPD) and, 65–66
Sexual function (female), 111–119. *See also* Libido; Menopause

  diagram of reproductive system, Plate 5
  estrogen replacement and, 141
  hysterectomies and, 153
  testosterone and, 115
Sexual function (male), 92–110. *See also* Libido
  depression and, 103
  diagram of reproductive system, Plate 6
  hormonal system and, 102–103
  injectable drugs, 108–110
  intermittent problems with, 106–107
  medications and, 104–110
  nervous system and, 100–102
  penile implants, 110
  tri-mix for, 109
  TURP (transurethral resection of prostate) and, 160
  vacuum pumps for, 110
  vascular system and, 94–100
Sexual relations, 89–119. *See also* Libido; Sexual function (female); Sexual function (male)
  exercise and, 38
  fertility issues and, 130
  food and, 198
  health benefits of, 93
  meditation and, 249
  men's issues, 92–110
  obesity and, 190
  oral sex, 99
  pheromones and, 118
  stress and, 101
  vascular system and, 94–100
  women's issues, 111–119
Sheehy, Gail, 9, 114
Sibutramine, 195
Sickle-cell anemia, 97
Sick sinus syndrome, 23, Plate 3
Siegel, Bernie, 54
Sildenofil. *See* Viagra
Sinoatrial node, 19, Plate 2, Plate 3
  sick sinus syndrome, 23
Skin
  estrogen replacement and, 141
  sun damage and, 170–171
Skin cancers, 170–172
  illustrations of, Plate 8

283

Sleep. *See also* Insomnia
  sexual relations and, 93
Slo-Niacin, 27
Smoking, 18, 203–204, 205–212
  back pain and, 240
  cancer and, 32
  depression and, 67
  fertility issues and, 130
  free radicals and, 175
  gastric ulcers and, 179
  health effects of, 50, 206
  osteoporosis and, 145, 149, 206
  pregnancy and, 126
  schizophrenia and, 65
  sexual function (female) and, 116–117
  sexual function (male) and, 94
  surgery and, 239
  vascular disease and, 29
  Zyban for, 209
Snacking, 200
Snoring, 191
Social isolation, 49
  health risks of, 71–72
Social support systems, 71–72
  for alcoholics, 213
  benefits of, 51
  physicians and, 59
  self-assessment, 78
  smoking cessation groups, 210
Solvay Laboratories, 147
Somaticizers, 55
Soybeans
  hot flashes and, 145
  oil, 181–182
Spermicidal foams, 129
  cervical cancer, prevention of, 136
Spider angiomas, 215
Spina bifida, 124, 128, 181
Spiritual life, 243–244. *See also* Meditation
  in Ananda, 259–262
  fertility and, 131
  goals for, 7
  Osler and, 245–246
  physicians assessing, 59
  recommendations for, 269
Squamous cell carcinomas, 170
  illustration, Plate 8
Stallone, Sylvester, 90
Statins, 27

Statistically significant studies, 177
Stomach cancer, 214
Stool samples, 168
Streptokinase, 163
Stress, 49. *See also* Meditation
  angina and, 19
  melatonin and, 186
  resistance to illness and, 69
  sexual relations and, 101
  somaticizers, 55
Strokes, 17, 25–26. *See also* Hemorrhagic stroke
  aspirin and, 179
  coronary bypass surgery and, 236–237
  omega-3 fatty acids and, 183
Sugar
  blues from, 47
  osteoporosis and, 145
Suicide
  contemplation of, 68
  meditation and, 248
Sun damage, 170–171
Superior vena cava, 19, Plate 3
Supplements, 173–188
  aspirin, 178–181
  DHEA (dehydroepiandrosterone), 184–185
  garlic, 183–184
  human growth hormone, 187–188
  melatonin, 186–187
  omega-3 fatty acids, 181–183
  recommendations for, 267
Surgery, 235–241. *See also* Coronary bypass surgery; Hysterectomies
  elective surgeries, 238
  mastectomy, 138
  meditation and, 241
  prostate surgery, 102
  vitamin C and healing, 239
Surgical menopause, 92
Swimming, 201
Sympathetic nervous system, 100–101
  meditation and, 248

T
Tagamet, 104
Tamoxifen, 138, 143
Television, 11

Tenaculum, 152
Terazosin, 106
Teresa, Mother, 264
Testicles, Plate 6
Testicular atrophy, 215
Testicular cancer, 161
Testosterone
  DHEA and, 185
  exercise and, 38
  female sexual desire and, 115
  sexual function (male) and, 95, 102–103
  sexual relations and, 93
  weight training and, 39
Thinning the blood. *See* Blood thinners
Thoracic aorta, Plate 1
Thorazine, 65
Thrombotic stroke, 25
Thyroid
  screening, 169
  weight loss and, 194
Thyroid-stimulating hormone (TSH), 169
Tissue plasminogen activator (TPA), 163
Tomatoes, prostate cancer and, 158
Tonsillectomies, 174
Touch
  healing and, 83–88
  physicians assessing, 59
Trazodone, 104–105
Triamterene, 104
Triplets, 127
Trisomies, 127–128
Tuberculosis, 18
Tuna, 47
Turkey, 46
TURP (transurethral resection of prostate), 160
T-waves, Plate 2
Twin births, 127
Tylenol, 178
Type I diabetes, 170
Type II diabetes, 170

U
University of California, Berkeley study, 74
University of Galveston Medical School study, 244–245
University of Massachusetts Medical Center study, 187

University of Western Ontario study, 187
Urinary tract, estrogen and, 141
Uterine cancer
  mortality rate, 155
  obesity and, 191
Uterus, 137, Plate 5. *See also* Hysterectomies
  endorphins and, 154

V
Vaccination recommendations, 268
Vacuum pumps, 110
Vagina, Plate 5
  estrogen creams and, 117
Vaginal artery, Plate 5
Vaillant, George, 9, 244
Valium
  sexual function (female) and, 117
  sexual function (male) and, 104
Van Houten, Peter, 260
Varicose veins, Plate 1
Vascular disease, 18–32. *See also* Heart attacks; Strokes
Vascular system
  sexual function (female) and, 116
  sexual function (male) and, 94–100
Vasomax, 100
Vegetables, 22
  prostate cancer and, 158
Vegetarian diet, 192–193
Ventricular fibrillation, 24

Verapamil, 106
Vertebral artery, Plate 4
Viagra, 92–93, 96–97, 108
Vicodin, 117
Visualization and heart disease, 257–258
Vitamin A as antioxidant, 175–176
Vitamin B, homocysteine levels and, 180
Vitamin B_3, 27
Vitamin B_6, 180
Vitamin B_{12}, 180
Vitamin C
  as antioxidant, 175, 176
  osteoporosis and, 145
  surgery and, 239
Vitamin D
  osteoporosis and, 145
  sun and, 170
Vitamin E
  as antioxidant, 175, 176
  hemorrhagic stroke and, 183
  prostate cancer and, 158
Vitamin K, osteoporosis and, 145

W
Walking, 48
Wallace, Robert Keith, 249
Warfarin. *See* Coumadin
Water, heart attack risk and, 20
Weight, 189–202. *See also* Obesity
  back pain and, 240
  blocks to losing, 67

  diet and, 46
  fertility issues and, 130
  human growth hormone and, 187
  methods for losing, 196–197
  thyroid and, 169
Weight training, 30
  weight loss and, 200
Wheat-germ oil, 181–182
Wilder, Gene, 135
Willis, Thomas, 28
Workaholics, 205
Work goals, 7
Wrinkles, 171

X
Xanax
  sexual function (female) and, 117
  sexual function (male) and, 104
X-chromosome, 116, 128
Xenical, 195
XXY syndrome, 128
XYY syndrome, 128

Y
Y-chromosome, 116, 128
Yoga
  heart disease and, 257–258
  osteoporosis and, 149
Yo-yo dieting, 199

Z
Zoloft, 104
  sexual function (male) and, 104
Zyban, 209

About the Author

Alan Bonsteel, M.D., has written and lectured extensively on health subjects, both for the general public and for other physicians. He sees patients in his clinic at Concord Family Practice in Clayton, California, and he is Director of the Emergency Department at Mercy Westside Hospital in Taft, California. He was formerly the Director of the Emergency Department at Southern Inyo District Hospital in Lone Pine, California (in the Owens Valley at the base of Mt. Whitney) and still works there part time. He is a graduate of Dartmouth Medical School and completed an internship at the University of California at Davis School of Medicine and a residency in family practice at the McGill School of Medicine in Montreal.

Dr. Bonsteel was born in 1951 in Los Angeles. He now lives in San Francisco with his wife and partner in creating this book, Chantal Charbonneau. In his spare time he plays ice hockey and campaigns for reform of America's public schools.